CRYSTAL
PRESCRIPTIONS

Volume 2

An A-Z guide to more than
1,250 conditions and their new
generation healing stones

CRYSTAL
PRESCRIPTIONS

Volume 2

An A-Z guide to more than
1,250 conditions and their new
generation healing stones

Judy Hall

Author of the best-selling
The Crystal Bible series

BOOKS

Winchester, UK
Washington, USA

JOHN HUNT PUBLISHING

First published by O-Books, 2014
O-Books is an imprint of John Hunt Publishing Ltd., 3 East St., Alresford,
Hampshire SO24 9EE, UK
office@jhpbooks.net
www.johnhuntpublishing.com

For distributor details and how to order please visit the 'Ordering' section on our
website.

A CIP catalogue record for this book is available from the British Library.

Design: Stuart Davies

UK: Printed and bound by CPI Group (UK) Ltd, Croydon, CR0 4YY
US: Printed and bound by Thomson-Shore, 7300 West Joy Road, Dexter, MI 48130

We operate a distinctive and ethical publishing philosophy
in all areas of our business, from our global network of
authors to production and worldwide distribution.

CONTENTS

Disclaimer

The information given in this directory is in no way intended to be a substitute for treatment by a medical practitioner. Further assistance should be sought from a suitably qualified crystal healer. Healing can be defined as bringing the body, emotions, mind and spirit back into energetic balance. It does not imply a cure.

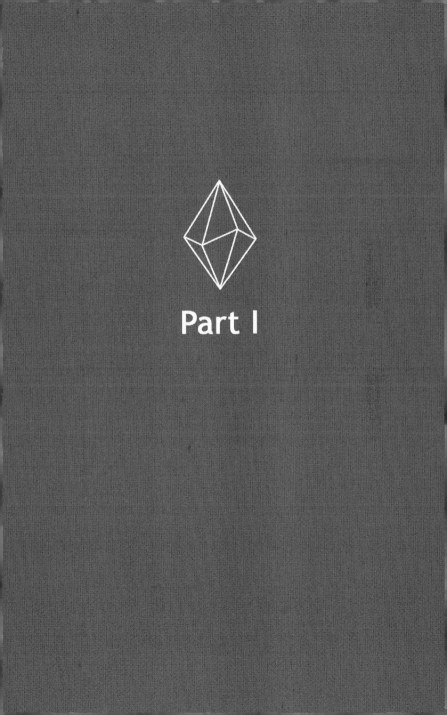

Part I

Crystal Preliminaries

Whether you are a newcomer to the crystal world or an experienced healer, this directory will help you to find exactly what you need for your healing work. The original *Crystal Prescriptions* covered crystals that were readily available at the time of writing, many of which dealt with physical symptoms. But the crystal world has moved on rapidly since then and more than 450 new crystals have come on to the market so a new volume is called for. It does not supersede the first volume. It is an adjunct to it. Many of these new generation stones have a higher vibration than those historically available. They rapidly raise awareness, lifting the frequency of the physical and subtle bodies, helping to assimilate an influx of higher vibrational energies and expanding awareness. Nevertheless, the new generation stones still have a practical healing application, although for some that healing takes place at a psychological, psyche or soul level.

The new high vibration crystals

In the last few years there has been an influx of exceptionally high vibration crystals that are harnessing the power of the highest dimensions to assist humankind to evolve. The frequency of these crystals is finer and lighter than those previously known. Where they really come into their own is in helping to bring about a vibrational shift of consciousness for the Earth and everyone on it. Literally taking us into a new dimension – or, rather, opening all possible dimensions. Indeed, there are many crystals becoming available now whose stated aim is to usher in a 'new age of awareness' of being both human and divine at one and the same time.

However, the crystals also point out that we cannot achieve this unity until we've done our own personal healing and growth work – with which they also assist. These new crystals didn't arrive with instructions for use (but you can use my book *The Crystal Experience* to learn how to tune in yourself). It's rather like having a totally new programme installed on a computer without operating instructions and then having to fathom out exactly how to utilise the enormous potential it offers. Fortunately I've been running crystal workshops that have attracted some very experienced crystal workers and 'beginners' who were eager to learn so we've explored that potential together and you can reap the benefit in this book.

Definition of healing

In the context of this book, disease or illness is a dis-ease, the final manifestation of spiritual, environmental, psychological, karmic, emotional, mental or physical imbalance or distress. Healing means bringing mind, body and spirit back into balance and facilitating evolution for the soul. It occurs at a subtle energetic level. It does not imply a cure.

What does this new directory do?

This directory is, as with volume 1, first and foremost a 'first-aid' guide to assist you to deal with specific issues. It lists conditions and matches them to the crystals that can heal them, whether the issue arises at a physical, emotional, mental or spiritual level. However, crystal healing does not deal primarily with specific conditions. Being a holistic system, it addresses dis-ease on more subtle levels, often bringing to light the underlying causes of a condition. This is particularly so when using the new generation high vibration stones as they rapidly clear blockages before realigning the whole system.

Why are so many more crystals included?

Well, apart from the fact that so many more crystals are now available, there are infinite possibilities to cover because every body is different. As I've said, crystal workers believe that the frequency of our planet and of our bodies is being raised. That our consciousness is expanding through multidimensions and that each person is at a unique and very personal stage of spiritual unfoldment and assimilation of the new vibrations. Therefore, different crystals are required depending on individual energetic frequencies. There are crystals to remove blockages and to adjust the physical and subtle bodies to facilitate the assimilation of the new vibrations, and also ones that take a fresh approach to old problems. Many of these crystals work from the spiritual level of being, having a subtle effect on the mental, emotional, psychic and physical bodies.

Crystals and the Chakras

The chakras are linkage points between your aura (the subtle bodies that form a biomagnetic sheath around your physical body) and your physical body. As with new crystals, additional chakras are becoming active to reach a higher energetic frequency. Each traditional chakra has its own colour but the new high vibration stones and higher chakras do not follow this colour association. The chakras below the waist are primarily physical, those in the upper torso are aligned to emotional issues that can create psychosomatic conditions, and those in the head function on a mental and intuitive basis, although the third eye, slightly above and between the eyebrows, the soma chakra above it and the crown chakras also function at a spiritual level, as do the higher crown chakras. Any imbalance, blockage or disturbance in these chakras creates discomfort that will ultimately manifest in your physical body but which can be restored to equilibrium before physical illness results.

When chakra imbalances are eliminated and the chakras are harmonized to work together, it leads to better health and a sense of well-being. It also assists in raising the frequency of your physical and subtle bodies so that you can access the multidimensions of consciousness and activate intercellular healing.

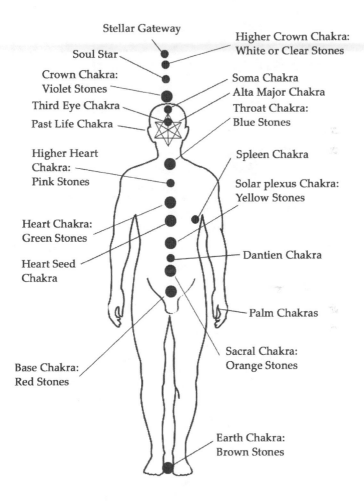

Stellar Gateway

Higher Crown Chakra: White or Clear Stones

Soul Star

Crown Chakra: Violet Stones

Soma Chakra

Alta Major Chakra

Third Eye Chakra

Throat Chakra: Blue Stones

Past Life Chakra

Higher Heart Chakra: Pink Stones

Spleen Chakra

Solar plexus Chakra: Yellow Stones

Heart Chakra: Green Stones

Heart Seed Chakra

Dantien Chakra

Palm Chakras

Base Chakra: Red Stones

Sacral Chakra: Orange Stones

Earth Chakra: Brown Stones

Crystals and the Chakras

Chakra Connections

Each chakra is connected to an area of life and to the physiology of the human body. Blockages or imbalances in a chakra create specific areas of physical, emotional, mental or spiritual dis-ease and personality traits or issues that can be brought back into balance and healed by placing the appropriate crystal on to the chakra (see page 13). If a chakra is out of balance – stuck open or blocked – it will lead to typical dis-eases as shown under each chakra. A constantly-open chakra is particularly vulnerable to influence from outside as there is no protection.

The Chakras

Earth Star (beneath your feet)
Area: Everyday reality and groundedness.
Physiology: The physical body, electrical systems of the body and the sensory organs.
Effect: Earth Star imbalances or blockages lead to discomfort in your physical body, feelings of helplessness and ungroundedness accompanied by an inability to function practically in the world. An out of balance Earth

Star picks up adverse environmental factors such as geopathic stress, 'black' ley lines and toxic pollutants. When this chakra is functioning well you are grounded and comfortable in incarnation.

Typical dis-eases are lethargic: ME, arthritis, cancer, muscular disorders, depression, psychiatric disturbances, autoimmune diseases.

Base (base of your spine/perineum)

Area: Basic survival instincts and security issues.

Physiology: Gonads, adrenals, veins, lower back, rectum, lower extremities, lymph system, skeleton system (teeth and bones), immune system, prostate gland, kidney, bladder and elimination system, sense of smell.

Effect: Imbalances in this chakra lead to sexual disturbances and feelings of anger, impotence and frustration. When it is functioning well you are confident and self-assertive.

Typical dis-eases are constant low level or flare up suddenly: stiffness in joints, chronic lower back pain, renal, reproductive or rectal disorders such as fluid retention/constipation (diarrhoea if stuck open), varicose veins or hernias, the extremes of bipolar disorder, glandular disturbances, personality and anxiety disorders, autoimmune diseases.

Sacral (navel) (slightly below your waist)

Area: Creativity, fertility and acceptance of yourself as a sexual being.

Physiology: Testes, ovaries, uterus, lumbar and pelvic region, spleen, large intestine, immune system, kidneys, gall bladder, bladder and elimination system, the sense of taste.

Effect: Imbalances in this chakra lead to infertility and blocked creativity. The sacral chakra is where 'hooks' from other people may make themselves felt, particularly from sexual encounters. When it is functioning well you are creative and enlivened.

Typical dis-eases are toxic and psychosomatic: PMT and muscle cramps, reproductive blockages or diseases, impotence, infertility, allergies, addictions, eating disorders, diabetes, liver or intestinal dysfunction – irritable bowel, chronic back pain, urinary infections.

Dantien: (on top of the sacral, just beneath navel)
Area: The powerpoint.

Physiology: Autonomic nervous and energy-conductive systems, regulation of the functioning of internal organs and involuntary processes such as breathing and heartbeat. Sensory impulses to the brain.

Effect: An adjunct to the sacral chakra and the point of balance for the physical body, the dantien is where Qi, life force, is stored and your body earthed. Blockages here mean that Qi cannot circulate efficiently and is not replenished. If the dantien is too open, energy is constantly drained. When it is functioning well you are energised and power-full.

Typical dis-eases relate to physical function and energy

utilisation: nervous system dysfunctions, autoimmune diseases, cardiac problems, high blood pressure, orthostatic hypotension, palpitations, adrenal overload, chronic fatigue, ME, Raynaud's, Parkinson's, digestive problems, diabetes, light-headedness, powerlessness, feeling ill at ease in incarnation.

Solar plexus (slightly above your waist)
Area: Emotional communication and assimilation.
Physiology: Pancreas, adrenals, stomach, liver, small intestine, digestion, metabolism, lymphatic system, skin, eyesight.
Effect: Blockages in the solar plexus can lead to taking on other people's feelings and problems, or to being overwhelmed by your own emotions. This chakra also affects energy utilisation. Emotional 'hooks' from other people can be found here. When it is functioning well you are emotionally balanced and caring.
Typical dis-eases are emotional and demanding: stomach ulcers, ME, 'fight or flight' adrenaline imbalances, insomnia and chronic anxiety, digestive problems, gallstones, pancreatic failure, eczema and other skin conditions, eating disorders and phobias.

Spleen (below left armpit)
Area: Assertion and empowerment.
Physiology: Pancreas, autoimmune and energy systems of the body.
Effect: If this chakra is imbalanced, you will have anger

issues or suffer constant irritation, with your body turning in to attack itself. If the chakra is too open, other people can draw on your energy, leaving you depleted particularly at the immune level. When it is functioning well you are invulnerable and able to assert yourself appropriately.

Typical dis-eases are psychosomatic and reactive: chronic fatigue, heart attacks, angina, chest infections, asthma, frozen shoulder, ulcers.

Heart seed (base of breastbone)
Area: Soul remembrance and universal love.
Physiology: Beyond the physical.
Effect: Blockages in this chakra lead to a sense of disconnection and alienation. When it is functioning well you remember that you are an eternal soul on a human journey and you become aware of being part of a greater whole.

Typical dis-eases are psycho-spiritual rather than physical.

Heart (over your heart)
Area: Love and nurturing.
Physiology: Thymus, heart, circulation, lungs, shoulders, chest, sense of touch.
Effect: If your heart chakra is blocked, love cannot flourish, feelings such as jealousy are common and there is enormous resistance to change. When it is functioning well you are able to show unconditional love and compassion.

Typical dis-eases arise from depletion and possessiveness: heart and blood disorders, arteriosclerosis, angina, lethargy, anaemia, low blood sugar.

Higher heart (thymus) (between the heart and the throat)
Area: Compassion and safety.
Physiology: The psychic and physical immune systems, lymphatic system, elimination and purification organs.
Effect: If this chakra is blocked, unconditional love and service cannot be offered. You will be emotionally needy and unable to express feelings openly. Your psychic and physical immune systems will not be able to function. If it is functioning well you are psychically and physically strong and feel safe in incarnation.
Typical dis-eases follow those of the heart, arteriosclerosis together with viral infections and immune system disorders, tinnitus, epilepsy.

Throat (the centre of your throat)
Area: Communication and self-expression.
Physiology: Thyroid, throat, tonsils, nose, sinuses, tongue, ears, respiratory system, nervous system, skin, speech and body language.
Effect: If this chakra is blocked, your thoughts and feelings cannot be verbalized. Other people's opinions can cause you difficulties. If it is functioning well you can express yourself clearly.
Typical dis-eases are active and block communication: sore

throat/quinsy, inflammation of trachea, sinus, constant colds and viral infections, tinnitus and ear infections, jaw pain and gum disease, tooth problems (relate to root beliefs), thyroid imbalances, high blood pressure, ADHD, autism, speech impediment, psychosomatic dis-eases such as irritable bowel.

Third eye (brow) (above and between your eyebrows)
Area: Intuition and mental connection.
Physiology: Pineal, brain, neurological system, sinuses, eyes, ears, scalp, hearing.
Effect: Imbalances in this chakra can create a sense of being bombarded by other people's thoughts, or lead to being overtaken by wild and irrational intuitions that have no basis in truth. Controlling or coercing mental 'hooks' from other people can lock in and affect your thoughts. If it is functioning well you will be intuitive and have acute mental clarity.
Typical dis-eases are intuitive and metaphysical: migraines, mental overwhelm, schizophrenia, cataracts, iritis and other eye problems, epilepsy, autism, spinal and neurological disorders, sinus and ear infections, high blood pressure, 'irritations' of all kinds.

Soma chakra (above the third eye, at the hairline)
Area: Spiritual connection.
Physiology: The connection point between the subtle energetic systems and the physical, etheric and light bodies.

Effect: This chakra is where your subtle bodies, including the lightbody, attach themselves to the physical. When this chakra is stuck open it is all too easy for discarnate spirits to attach or for you to float out of your physical body. If it is functioning well you can safely explore the spiritual dimensions of life.

Typical dis-eases are autistic and disconnected or dyspraxic and may include Down's syndrome, autism and ADHD, chronic fatigue, delusional states.

Past life (behind your ears, along the bony ridge)
Area: Memory and hereditary issues.
Physiology: DNA, genetic and cellular memory.
Effect: Imbalances here mean that you are stuck in the past and cannot move forward, and may well be repeating personal past life or ancestral patterns passed down through your family. If it is functioning well you can draw on your karmic and ancestral wisdom to negotiate life.

Typical dis-eases are deeply ingrained and may be genetically based: chronic illnesses, especially immune or endocrine deficiencies, genetic or physical malfunctions.

Crown (top of your head)
Area: Spiritual communication and awareness.
Physiology: Pituitary, hypothalamus, brain, spine, central nervous system, hair, subtle energy bodies.
Effect: If the crown chakra is blocked, attempting to control others is common; and if it is stuck open,

obsession and openness to spiritual interference or possession can result. If it is functioning well you express yourself as a spiritual being and attain unity consciousness.

Typical dis-eases arise out of disconnection: metabolic syndrome, 'unwellness' with no known cause, nervous system disturbances, electromagnetic and environmental sensitivity, depression, dementia, ME, insomnia or excessive sleepiness, 'biological clock' disturbances such as jet lag.

Soul Star (a foot above the head)

Area: Service and spiritual enlightenment.

Physiology: The subtle energetic systems of the body and the lightbody.

Effect: If this chakra is stuck open, you will be spaced out and open to delusion. Influence from other realms and entity attachment is possible. If this chakra is appropriately open there is a connection to higher realms, spiritual guidance and multidimensions.

Typical dis-eases are spiritual rather than physical.

Stellar Gateway (two feet above the head)

Area: The multidimensional cosmic portal.

Physiology: The subtle energetic systems of the body and lightbody.

Effect: If this chakra is blocked or stuck open low-level entities can attach and disseminate spiritual disinformation leading to delusions. If this chakra is appropriately open there is a connection to higher realms and multidimensions.

Typical dis-eases are spiritual rather than physical.

Alta Major (Ascension Chakra) (inside the skull, the access point is at the base of the skull)

Area: Accelerating and expanding consciousness.

Physiology: The subtle and physical endocrine systems, hippocampus, hypothalamus, pineal and pituitary glands; brain function, the cerebellum and voluntary muscle movements, the medulla oblongata controlling breathing, heart rate and blood pressure; occipital area and the optic nerve, throat, spine, sleeping patterns.

Effect: This chakra contains your past life karma and the contractual agreements you made before incarnating. It stretches from the base of the skull to the crown connecting the past life and soma chakras, hippocampus, hypothalamus, pineal and pituitary glands with the third eye, throat and the higher crown chakras. If the alta major is functioning well your consciousness expands to encompass other dimensions and your subtle endocrine system harmonizes the subtle bodies with the physical, opening your intuition. You will have a strong sense of direction in life.

Typical dis-eases are ancestral, karmic or those of disorientation: metabolic dysfunction, eye problems, floaters, cataracts, migraines, headaches and feelings of confusion, 'dizziness' or 'floatiness', loss of sense of purpose and spiritual depression, fear, terror, adrenaline rush.

Finding Your Prescription

The best way to select your crystals is to choose them intuitively, to dowse for them (see pages 26/27), or to utilise what you already have in your crystal toolkit.

Most entries in this directory offer a choice of crystals to assist a particular condition or issue. While all the stones listed could potentially help you, selecting the right crystal is crucial if you are to obtain maximum benefit and the fastest relief. Some crystals have a much finer vibration than others, working from the etheric or karmic blueprint to adjust the physical, and some work at a physical level. Others operate more subtly, frequently bringing underlying causes to the surface so that you may need to use a series of crystals.

You may find that you are instinctively drawn to a particular stone and it may be one that you already have in your collection. If so, try this one first. You can also dowse when purchasing a healing crystal, either by allowing your fingers instinctively to pick the right stone from a number of stones – usually the one that 'sticks' to them – or using a pendulum or finger dowsing (see pages 26/27).

Dowsing is an excellent way to select your crystal(s)

and you can either use a pendulum for this purpose or finger dowse. Both methods use the ability of your intuitive body-mind connection to tune into subtle vibrations and to influence your hands. A focused mind, trust in the process, carefully worded questions and a clear intent will support your dowsing and your healing.

Dowsing

Framing your question

Framing your question with precision is essential if you are to achieve the most beneficial result. Your questions need to be unambiguous and capable of a straight 'yes' or 'no' answer. They also need to be asked with serious intent. An irresponsible approach or a frivolous question is unlikely to reveal anything of lasting benefit and could actually do harm as crystals are powerful tools that pick up and amplify your thoughts. They should be treated with respect.

Take time to prepare yourself to ask the question. Sit quietly for a few moments, bringing your focus away from the outside world and quietening your mind. Word your question carefully. If, for instance, you ask: 'Is this the right crystal for me?', the answer could well be 'yes' but it may not refer to the condition you wish to relieve at that precise moment. It could indicate a crystal that would give you long-term benefit for an, as yet, unrecognized issue that exists at an emotional, mental or soul level. That crystal could well be of value to you in the long term, but it would not heal the immediate symptom.

You need to be specific. If you are finger dowsing (see pages 26/27), ask: 'Is [name of crystal] the best and most appropriate crystal to treat my headache at this time?' If you are pendulum dowsing (see page 27), ask: 'Please show me the best and most appropriate crystal to treat my headache now.' It can also be worthwhile enquiring: 'Is there a deeper condition underlying my symptom?' If the answer is 'yes', you can ask: 'Does this condition lie at the physical [wait for a moment for the pendulum to respond], emotional [wait for a moment], mental [wait for a moment] or soul [wait for a moment] level?' You can then put your finger on each letter in the directory in turn. When you find a 'yes' response, run your finger down the page until the pendulum locates the underlying cause of your dis-ease.

Finger Dowsing

Finger dowsing answers 'yes' and 'no' questions quickly and unambiguously, and can be done unobtrusively in situations where a pendulum might provoke unwanted attention. This method of dowsing works particularly well for people who are kinaesthetic, that is to say their body responds intuitively to subtle feelings, but anyone can learn to finger dowse.

To finger dowse

To finger dowse, hold the thumb and first finger of your right hand together (see illustration). Loop the thumb and finger of your left hand through to make a 'chain'. Ask your question clearly and unambiguously – you can speak it aloud or keep it within your mind. Now pull gently but firmly. If the chain breaks, the answer is 'no'. If it holds, the answer is 'yes'.

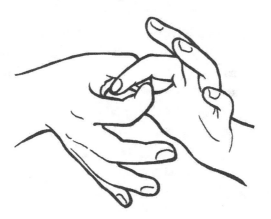

Finger dowsing

Pendulum

If you are familiar with pendulum dowsing, use the pendulum in your usual way. If you are not, this skill is easily learned.

To pendulum dowse

To pendulum dowse, hold your pendulum between the thumb and forefinger of your most receptive hand with about a hand's breadth of chain hanging down to the pendulum – you will soon learn what is the right length for you. Wrap the remaining chain around your fingers so that it does not obstruct the dowsing.

You will need to ascertain which is a 'yes' and which a 'no' response. Some people find that the pendulum swings in one direction for 'yes' and at right angles to that axis for 'no', while others have a backwards and forwards swing for one reply, and a circular motion for the other. A 'wobble' of the pendulum can indicate a 'maybe' or that it is not appropriate to dowse at that time, or that the wrong question is being asked. In which case, ask if it is appropriate and, if the answer is 'yes', check that you are framing the question in the correct way. If the pendulum stops completely it is usually inappropriate to ask at that time.

You can ascertain your particular pendulum response by holding the pendulum over your knee and asking: 'Is my name [correct name]?' The direction that the pendulum swings will indicate 'yes'. Check by asking: 'Is my name [incorrect name]?' to establish 'no'. Or, you can programme in 'yes' and 'no' by swinging the pendulum in a particular direction a few times, saying as you do: 'This is yes' and swinging it in a different direction to programme in 'no'.

To ascertain the best crystal for you

To ascertain which crystal will be most beneficial for you, hold the pendulum in your most receptive hand. Put the forefinger of your other hand on the condition or issue. Slowly run your finger along the list of possible crystals, noting whether you get a 'yes' or 'no' response. Check the whole list to see which 'yes' response is strongest as there may well be several that would be appropriate or you may need to use several crystals in combination. Another way to do this, if you have several of the crystals available, is to touch each crystal in turn, again noting the 'yes' or 'no' response.

If you get a 'no' response when checking out the condition, touch each of the capital letters in turn until you receive a 'yes', then run your finger down the conditions. This may well reveal something that underlies the apparent issue.

How long should I use a crystal?

A pendulum can also be used to establish for how long a crystal should be left in place. This is particularly useful if you are placing the crystal over an organ or around your body or bed, but it can also be helpful if you are wearing a crystal and need to know whether or not to wear it at night – in which case you will get a 'yes' or 'no' answer to the question: 'Should I remove this crystal at night?' To establish timing, use an arc on which you have marked five-minute or one-hour or one-day intervals (ask in advance whether the period should be checked in minutes, hours or days). Hold the hand with the pendulum over the centre of the arc and ask that the pendulum will go towards the correct period (see illustration).

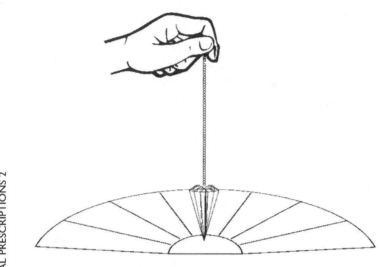

Dowsing over an Arc

Purifying and Focusing Your

Crystals

Purifying Your Crystal

As crystals hold the energetic charge of everyone who comes into contact with them and absorb emanations from their surroundings, as well as your personal energies, they need regular purifying. This is particularly so when they are being used for healing. It is sensible to purify and re-energize a crystal every time it is used. The method employed will depend on the type of crystal. Soft and friable crystals, for instance, and those that are attached to a base can be damaged by water, and soft stones such as Halite will dissolve. These are best purified by a 'dry' process such as brown rice or sunlight, but sturdier crystals benefit from being placed under running water or in the sea.

Crystals work best when their energy is harnessed and focused with intent towards the task at hand as this activates them. By taking the time to attune a crystal to your own unique frequency, you enhance its vibratory effect and amplify its healing power.

Methods:

Running water

Hold your crystals under a running tap, or pour bottled water over them, or place them in a stream or the ocean to draw off negative energy (use a bag to hold small crystals). You can also immerse appropriate crystals in a bowl of water into which a handful of sea salt or rock salt has been added. (Salt is best avoided if the crystal is layered or friable.) Dry the crystal carefully afterwards and place in the sun to re-energize.

Rice or salt

Place your crystal in a bowl of salt or brown rice and leave overnight for the negative energies to be absorbed. (Brush salt off carefully and make sure that it has been removed from any niches or cracks in the crystal as otherwise it will absorb water in the future and could cause splintering.) Place the crystals in the sun to re-energize.

Smudging

Sage, sweetgrass or joss sticks are excellent for smudging as they quickly remove negative energies. Light the smudge stick and pass it over the crystal if it is large, or hold the crystal in your hand in the smoke if it is small. It is traditional to fan the smoke gently with a feather but this is not essential.

Visualizing light

Hold your crystal in your hands and visualize a column of bright white light coming down and covering the crystal, absorbing anything negative it may have picked up and restoring the pure energy once more. If you find visualization difficult, you can use the light of a candle.

Crystal clearing essences

A number of crystal clearing essences are available from flower essence suppliers, crystal shops and the Internet (see Resources). You can either drop the essence directly on to the crystal, gently rubbing it over the crystal with your finger, or put a few drops into clean spring water in an atomiser or spray bottle and gently mist the crystal.

Re-Energizing Your Crystal

Crystals can be placed on a Quartz cluster or on a large Carnelian to re-energize them but the light of the sun is an excellent energizer. Red and yellow crystals particularly enjoy being placed in the sun, and white and pale-coloured crystals respond well to the moon. (Be aware that sunlight focused through a crystal can be a fire hazard and delicate crystals will lose their colour quickly if left exposed to light.) Some brown crystals such as Smoky Quartz respond to being placed on or in the earth. If you bury a crystal, remember to mark its position clearly.

Focusing and Activating Your Crystal

Once your crystal has been purified and re-energized, sit quietly holding the crystal in your hands for a few minutes until you feel in tune with it. Picture it surrounded by light and love. State that the crystal is dedicated to the highest good of all who use it. Then state very clearly your intention for the crystal – that it will heal or protect you, for instance. If it is intended for a specific purpose such as healing a particular condition, state that also. Repeat the intention several times to anchor it into the crystal.

Crystal Essences

Crystal essences are an excellent way to use the healing power of crystals, and several crystals can be combined provided you dowse to check compatibility. The essences are ideally suited to children as they can be gently rubbed on the skin or sprayed into a room. Essences intended for adult use are usually added to a glass of water and sipped, or taken from a dropper bottle, or sprayed around the aura or environment.

Crystal essences are made by transferring the subtle energies and minute concentrations of the mineral constituents of the crystal into water, which then stores the vibrations and transfers them to the physical or subtle bodies in exactly the same way that a homoeopathic remedy works. The essence is bottled and a preservative – brandy, vodka or cider vinegar – added. If the essence is to be taken by those for whom alcohol is inappropriate, cider vinegar can be used as a preservative.

Caution: Some stones may contain trace minerals that are toxic (see the list in Contraindications), and essences from these stones need to be made by an indirect method that transfers the vibrations without transferring any of the toxic material from the stone (see page 88). If in doubt, make the essence by the indirect method, which is also suitable for fragile or layered stones. Always wash your hands after handling one of these stones and use a tumbled version wherever possible.

Making a Crystal Essence

You will need the appropriate crystal, which has been cleansed and purified (see pages 31–34), one or two clean glass bowls, spring water and a suitable bottle in which to keep the essence (coloured glass is preferable to clear as it preserves the vibrations better). Essences can be made by the direct or indirect method. Spring water should be used rather than tap water that has chlorine, fluoride and aluminium added to it. Water from a spring with healing properties is particularly effective.

Direct method

Place enough spring water in a glass bowl to just cover the crystal. Stand the bowl in sunlight for several hours. (If the bowl is left outside, cover with a glass lid or cling film to prevent insects falling into it.) If appropriate, the bowl can also be left overnight in moonlight.

Indirect method

If the crystal is toxic or fragile (see Contraindications page 88) place the crystal in a small glass bowl and stand the bowl within a large bowl that has sufficient spring water to raise the level above the crystal in the inner bowl. Stand the bowl in sunlight for several hours. (If the bowl is left outside, cover with a glass lid or cling film.) If appropriate, the bowl can also be left overnight in moonlight.

Bottling and preserving

If the essence is not to be used within a day or two, top up with two-thirds brandy, vodka, white rum or cider vinegar to one-third essence, otherwise the essence will become musty. This makes a 'mother tincture' that can be further diluted. To make a small dosage bottle, add seven drops of the mother essence to a dosage bottle containing two-thirds brandy and one-third water. If a spray bottle is being made, add seven drops of mother essence to pure water if using immediately. For prolonged use, vodka or white rum makes a useful preservative as it has no smell.

Using a crystal essence

For short-term use, an essence can be sipped every few minutes or rubbed on the affected part. Hold the water in your mouth for a few moments. If a dropper bottle has been made, drop seven drops under your tongue at regular intervals until the symptoms or condition ceases.

Essences can also be applied to the skin, either at the wrist or over the site of a problem, or added to bath water.

If a spray bottle is made, spray all around the aura or

around the room. This is particularly effective for clearing negative energies, especially from the crystals themselves, or from a sickroom or an electromagnetically or emotionally stressed place.

Using This Directory

In the directory you will find an A–Z list of symptoms and common issues that may occur physically, emotionally, mentally or spiritually with their appropriate healing crystals. Most entries have several crystals listed that would be beneficial, although a few have only one. There is a choice because everyone is subtly different and deeper causes may underlie a symptom. Crystals heal holistically – that is to say they work at a causal level on the whole person. What works for you will not necessarily work for your friend because you will have different causes for your dis-ease and you may well have different body types. Many of the entries also have a chakra or chakras associated with them. This means that the condition can be treated through putting appropriate stones on the chakra and leaving in place for 15–20 minutes or so.

To identify the right crystal, check out your symptom, condition or issue, and dowse or intuit which one(s) is/are appropriate. If you have several issues, you may well find that one crystal is beneficial for all. This will be the crystal for you. It could be that you already own a crystal, having been instinctively drawn to it. But you may be left with a choice of several crystals, in which case turn to page 24 to learn how to identify the one that will be of greatest benefit to you, although many crystals work well in combination. Occasionally certain crystals are contraindicated and you will find these listed in the directory under Contraindications (page 88).

Using your crystals for healing

Many of the directory entries indicate a chakra link through which a condition can be healed or you can dowse for or intuit this (see page 14 for further information on the physiology of the chakras). Most new generation and high vibration crystals can be placed over clothing on the chakra, over organs or the site of dis-ease and left in place for 15–20 minutes or so. They can also be

placed around the body, out in the aura or in your space to create energetic grids. Some are particularly beneficial when placed directly on the skin as they carry the energetic resonance of their mineral components. Crystals can also be taped in place, or worn for much longer periods for healing or prevention; or they can be kept in a pocket, or placed around your bed or a room.

If your crystal has a point, place it point towards yourself, or point down if placed on your body, to draw healing or re-energizing properties into your body. Place it point out, or point down below your feet to draw off toxic residues or emotional debris. Crystals are most effective when you are in a relaxed state and you need to be comfortable. If lying on your back is uncomfortable, for instance, and is not alleviated by placing a pillow under your knees, by all means sit in a chair. The stones can always be held or taped in place.

When you have placed the stones, close your eyes and breathe gently and evenly and allow yourself to relax and feel the energy of the crystal radiating out through your whole being.

You can also apply crystal essences (see pages 35–38). These essences convey crystal vibes to the body at a subtle level and are particularly effective for emotional conditions and for assimilating high vibrational downloads and making soul shifts.

Healing challenge

Occasionally crystal healing will trigger a 'healing challenge' when the symptoms appear to get worse rather than better and flu-like symptoms may occur. This is an indication of physical, emotional or mental toxins leaving the body and is all part of the body holistically healing itself. It occurs particularly in stress-related or chronic conditions. It can be soothed and facilitated by crystals such as Smoky Elestial Quartz, Eye of the Storm or Quantum Quattro and by drinking plenty of water (Shungite-infused water is ideal). If a healing challenge occurs use these stones for a few days until the symptoms dissipate and then return to the crystals you were using – having dowsed or intuited if they are still necessary.

Crystal consultations

Maybe an example or two will help here. Under current EU regulations, I cannot claim that a crystal 'cures' but I am allowed to share anecdotal experiences with you so I'll begin with one of my own. Having had pneumonia several times in the past, a cold or flu could be lethal but I cannot avoid the crowded places where viruses and bacteria thrive. Fortunately Shungite came to my rescue. Immersed in water for 48 hours, research has shown that it transforms the water into a biologically active life-enhancing substance, removing harmful microorganisms and pollutants. The research shows that Shungite absorbs pesticides, free radicals, viruses, bacteria and the like. Boosting physical well-being, it has a powerful effect on the immune system. I drink two litres of Shungite water every day (the Shungite is suspended in a bag in my filter jug, constantly charging up the water with crystal energy). In the three years I have been using this method, I have caught only one cough virus and that was mild. I also wear Shungite over my thymus (higher heart chakra) and have placed it around my computer to protect me from electromagnetic frequencies, which used to deplete me but no longer do so as the Shungite shields me.

You could place Shungite on your Earth Star to protect you from vibrational emissions, radiation, geopathogens and geopathic stress and the dis-eases these can create. Or, place it on your computer, or over your higher heart chakra, to shield you if you are electro-sensitive. But it has also been shown to be antioxidant, antibacterial, anti-inflammatory and antihistaminic. It energetically assists cellular metabolism, neurotransmitters, enzyme production, sore throats, burns, cardiovascular diseases, blood disorders, blood pressure, allergies, asthma, gastric disturbances, diabetes, arthritis, AIDS, cancer, osteoarthritis, kidney and liver disorders, gall-bladder dysfunction, autoimmune diseases, pancreatic disorders, impotence and chronic fatigue syndrome. A useful 'cure-all', Shungite strengthens the autoimmune, digestive and filtration systems of the body, and provides pain relief,

Another example I can share with you is a young woman who was desperate to conceive a baby. She had been trying for three years. As her sacral chakra was blocked and she had issues around her self-worth, I gave her a Menalite to place over her sacral chakra and to keep under her pillow at night. She conceived within a couple of days. Coincidence? I don't think so as she wasn't the first person to do so. She now has a beautiful baby boy. Menalite is traditionally used for birth. One of my clients mentioned she had had a really difficult first birth and was experiencing a challenging second pregnancy. So I gave her a Menalite to assist the pregnancy and the delivery. She reported that she held it throughout and felt hugely comforted and relaxed, and had an easy birth. She then gave it on to one of her friends who also benefitted. It is now being passed on from expectant mother to another.

With its powerful link to fertility and the feminine,

Menalite placed over a blocked base or sacral chakra energetically maintains hormonal balance, assisting puberty, pre-menstrual tension, menopausal symptoms, loss of libido and disorders of the male or female reproductive system.

Healing layouts

Crystals are very effective when laid out in grids, simple patterns that encompass, purify, generate and amplify energy. They can be used for personal or space healing or clearing.

Chakra layout

A very simple but effective layout is to place a cleansed and activated crystal over each of your chakras – you can dowse or intuit which crystals are suitable and which of the minor chakras should be included (see diagram on page 13). Begin with your feet and lay one below and between them, then place the crystals over the chakras moving up your body and slowly lying down as you do so. Finally place one or more at the top of your head. Lie still for about fifteen minutes and then gather up the crystals in the reverse order that you laid them down – i.e. beginning with the one(s) above your head. When you reach the crystal beneath your feet, place your hands on it for a few moments to ground your energy before getting up.

Crystal grids

Placing crystals in a geometric pattern around your body creates an energetic net that purifies, heals and rejuvenates your energies, bringing in harmony and well-being. Placing them around your space in a grid cleanses and protects the environment. Place the crystals at the points of the geometric figures. After you have laid out the crystal grid, join up the points with a wand or long-point crystal such as a Lemurian Seed.

Triangulation

Crystals: 3 cleansed and activated crystals

Lay one crystal above your head or centrally along a wall. Position the other two at the points of the triangle below your feet or in each corner of the room. Connect the points with a wand to strengthen the grid. Protective triangulation neutralizes negative energy and brings in positive well-being. This layout is particularly helpful placed around your bed.

Zigzag

Crystals: 8 or more cleansed and activated crystals

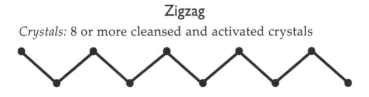

This layout is particularly helpful for sick building syndrome or to counteract environmental pollution. It also pulls energy up from the Earth to ground you, or draws down spiritual energy from the higher crown chakras. You can adjust the number of stones to fit the space. Lay in a zigzag pattern so that the crystals touch the walls on either side or are placed on either side of your body. Remember to cleanse the crystals regularly.

Pentangle

Crystals: 5 cleansed and activated stones

This layout is particularly useful for protection or for calling in healing and love. It enhances energy. Place the first crystal at the top and then follow the lines to place the remainder. Remember to join all the points with a wand to complete the circuit.

Star of David

Crystals: 6 cleansed and activated crystals
A traditional protection layout, placing the first triangle

point down and joining the points traps negative

energies for transmutation. Lay the second triangle over the top and join the points to draw in beneficial energy. The Star of David can also be used to draw in abundance and beneficial energies, in which case lay the first triangle point up to draw in the energies and place the second triangle point down to lock them in place.

Figure of eight

Crystals:
3 cleansed and activated high vibration stones such as new generation Quartzes
3 cleansed and activated grounding stones (see page 115)
1 synthesizing stone such as Elestial Quartz, Polychrome Jasper or Shiva Lingam
*turn to face upwards if possible

Drawing high vibration energy down into the body, the figure of eight layout synthesizes it with earth energy drawn up from the feet to create equilibrium and ground the raised vibrations. It creates core energy solidity that enables riding out energetic changes. Place the joining stone just below your navel or at the centre of the layout. Place a high vibration crystal at shoulder level, or halfway up the upper side, one at the top of your head or of the layout, and one halfway down the next side. Place a grounding stone level with your knees or halfway down the lower portion, then one beneath your feet or at the base of the layout, and the final one level with the one at your knees. Remember to complete the circuit back to the first stone placed.

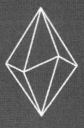

Part II
Directory of Conditions

- A -

Abandonment, overcome feelings of: Cassiterite, Chalcanthite, Quantum Quattro, Rhodozaz, Tugtupite. *Chakra:* base, heart

Abdomen: Anthrophyllite, Bastnasite, Smoky Amethyst. *Chakra:* sacral

Abdominal distension or colic: Crinoidal Limestone, Leopardskin Jasper. *Chakra:* sacral, dantien

Abortion, healing after: Menalite. *Chakra:* sacral

Absorption of nutrients: see Assimilation page 56

Abuse: Apricot Quartz, Azeztulite with Morganite, Eilat Stone, Honey Opal, Lazurine, Lemurian Jade, Pink Crackle Quartz, Proustite, Red Quartz, Septarian, Smoky Amethyst, Smoky Citrine, Xenotine. *Chakra:* base, sacral

> **break away from:** Xenotine. *Chakra:* sacral and solar plexus
>
> **emotional:** Apricot Quartz, Azeztulite with Morganite, Honey Opal, Lazurine, Mount Shasta Opal, Rosophia, Smoky Rose Quartz, Tugtupite, Xenotine. *Chakra:* sacral, heart
>
> **sexual:** Apricot Quartz, Eilat Stone, Proustite, Shiva Lingam. *Chakra:* base, sacral

Academic study: Anthrophyllite, Datolite, Diopside, Realgar and Orpiment, Tiffany Stone. *Chakra:* third eye

Acceptance of physical body: Celestobarite, Empowerite, Keyiapo, Llanite (Llanoite), Riebekite with

Sugilite and Bustamite, Schalenblende, Thompsonite and see Incarnation page 125. *Chakra:* earth star, base, dantien, crown

Accepting oneself: see Self-acceptance page 179

Accident prone: Black Moonstone (wear constantly)

Aches and pains: Blue Euclase, Cathedral Quartz, Hemimorphite, Quantum Quattro, Rhodozite (place over site).

Acid:

    acid/alkaline imbalance: Diaspore (Zultanite), Diopside, Gabbro, Klinoptilolith, Nunderite

    correct overacidification: Bornite, Bronzite, Diaspore (Zultanite), Kimberlite, Klinoptilolith

    acidosis/indigestion: Cryolite, Steatite

Acne: Snakeskin Agate (bathe in crystal essence)

Acupressure/Acupuncture: Halite, Preseli Bluestone

Addictions: Amethyst Elestial Quartz, Brandenberg Amethyst, Crackled Fire Agate, Fenster Quartz, Golden Selenite, Lazulite, Smoky Amethyst, Tantalite, Vera Cruz Amethyst. *Chakra:* base, sacral, dantien (or take as alcohol-free essence or carry at all times)

Addictive behaviour: Sichuan Quartz, Xenotine. *Chakra:* base, dantien

ADHD (Attention deficit disorder): Amblygonite, Brandenberg Amethyst, Cumberlandite, Lepidocrosite, Stichtite, Tantalite, Tanzine Aura Quartz. *Chakra:* dantien (or place in pocket)

Unless otherwise directed, apply crystal over organ or site of symptom, place on appropriate chakra, wear as jewellery, bathe with or take as a crystal essence.

Adrenals: Axinite, Epidote, Eye of the Storm, Gaspeite, Nunderite, Picrolite, Richterite. *Chakra:* base, dantien, solar plexus

    calming: Cacoxenite, Eye of the Storm, Jamesonite, Richterite

    stimulating: Fiskenaesset Ruby

Adverse environmental factors: Champagne Aura Quartz, Elestial Smoky Quartz, Ethiopian Opal, Khutnohorite, Petrified Wood, Shungite, Smoky Amethyst, Trummer Jasper. *Chakra:* earth star, dantien (place crystal at four corners of house or site, on computer etc.)

Aggression, ameliorate: Blizzard Stone, Fluorapatite, Pyrite in Magnesite. *Chakra:* base, dantien

Aging process, slow: Eisenkiesel

AIDS: see HIV page 121

Akashic Record: see page 160

Alcohol, mitigate effects of: Amethyst Elestial Quartz (use as alcohol-free crystal essence or carry stone)

Alcoholism: Amethyst Elestial Quartz, Vera Cruz Amethyst and see Addictions page 51. *Chakra:* base

Alienation, overcome: Amphibole Quartz, Bustamite with Sugilite, Champagne Aura Quartz, Gaia Stone. *Chakra:* earth star, solar plexus, soma

Align:

    physical, emotional, mental subtle bodies: Aurichalcite, Empowerite, Fulgarite, Golden

---

Unless otherwise directed, apply crystal over organ or site of symptom, place on appropriate chakra, wear as jewellery, bathe with or take as a crystal essence.

Coracalcite, Herderite, Lemurian Seed, Mount Shasta Opal, Nuummite, Paraiba Tourmaline, Schalenblende, Scheelite, Sillimanite, Thompsonite. *Chakra:* alta major (base of skull), soma

mind-body-spirit: Aurichalcite, Golden Coracalcite, Larvikite, Sillimanite. *Chakra:* alta major (base of skull)

the chakras: Annabergite, Barite, Black Kyanite, Gaia Stone, Lepidocrosite, Lemurian Seed, Paraiba Tourmaline, Picrolite, Sichuan Quartz, Sillimanite, and see pages 76–82. *Chakra:* earth star to higher crown, dantien

Alimentary canal: Eclipse Stone, Goethite (place on abdomen)

Allergies: Bastnasite, Bumble Bee Jasper, Golden Danburite, Shungite, Stone of Dreams. *Chakra:* higher heart (or carry crystal)

to animals: Poppy Jasper, Shungite

multiple chemical: Hackmanite, Shungite

Alta Major Chakra: see Chakras page 62

Altitude sickness: Aztee, Green Siberian Quartz, Sonora Sunrise

Alzheimer's: Eudialyte. *Chakra:* third eye

Amnesia: Revelation Stone. *Chakra:* crown

Anaemia: Cinnabar in Jasper, Cryolite, Goethite, Green Ridge Quartz, Limonite, Reinerite, Specularite, Tangerine Sun Aura Quartz. *Chakra:* heart, spleen

---

Unless otherwise directed, apply crystal over organ or site of symptom, place on appropriate chakra, wear as jewellery, bathe with or take as a crystal essence.

Analytic ability: Diopside, Eclipse Stone, Scapolite, Schalenblende, and see Mind page 147

Anaphylactic shock: Ouro Verde, Richterite, Tantalite. *Chakra:* dantien, heart, higher heart

Ancestral:

> **DNA:** Datolite, Eye of the Storm, Icicle Calcite, Petrified Wood, Pyrite in Quartz, Snakeskin Pyrite. *Chakra:* past life, alta major (base of skull)
>
> **line, healing:** Brandenberg Amethyst, Candle Quartz, Chlorite Quartz, Crinoidal Limestone, Datolite, Fairy Quartz, Ilmenite, Lemurian Aquitane Calcite, Mohawkite, Prasiolite, Rainforest Jasper, Shaman Quartz, Smoky Elestial Quartz, Spirit Quartz. *Chakra:* past life, base
>
> **issues:** Porphyrite (Chinese Letter Stone). *Chakra:* past life or alta major
>
> **patterns:** Anthrophyllite, Arfvedsonite, Celadonite, Candle Quartz, Crinoidal Limestone, Eclipse Stone, Garnet in Quartz, Glendonite, Green Ridge Quartz, Holly Agate, Mohawkite, Porphyrite (Chinese Letter Stone), Prasiolite, Rainbow Covellite, Rainbow Mayanite, Shaman Quartz with Chlorite, Scheelite, Starseed Quartz. *Chakra:* past life or alta major

Anger, ameliorate: Cinnabar in Jasper, Ethiopian Opal, Nzuri Moyo. *Chakra:* base, dantien

> **at god:** Eudialyte

Angina: Khutnohorite, Pyrite in Magnesite. *Chakra:* heart,

Unless otherwise directed, apply crystal over organ or site of symptom, place on appropriate chakra, wear as jewellery, bathe with or take as a crystal essence.

base

Animals: Dalmatian Stone

Anorexia: Azotic Topaz, Mystic Topaz, Picasso Jasper, Orange Kyanite, Tugtupite. *Chakra:* earth star, base, heart

Antibacterial: Blue Euclase, Cathedral Quartz, Honey Opal, Proustite, Shungite, Trummer Jasper (bathe in crystal essence, drink activated water or apply stone)

Anticarcinogenic: Champagne Aura Quartz, Klinoptilolith, Shungite

Antihistamine: Shungite

Anti-inflammatory: Greenlandite, Shungite. *Chakra:* base (or wear constantly)

Antioxidant: Diaspore (Zultanite), Khutnohorite, Klinoptilolith, Piemontite, Reinerite, Shungite, Tantalite

Antiseptic: Blue Euclase, Shungite (bathe in crystal essence or apply stone)

Antisocial behaviour: Blizzard Stone (place in environment)

Antispasmodic: Diopside, Chrome Diopside

Antiviral: Cathedral Quartz, Honey Opal, Quantum Quattro, Shaman Quartz, Shungite, Trummer Jasper. *Chakra:* higher heart

Anxiety: Galaxyite, Lemurian Aquitane Calcite, Lemurian Gold Opal, Khutnohorite, Nzuri Moyo, Oceanite, Owyhee Blue Opal, Pyrite in Magnesite, Riebekite with Sugilite and Bustamite, Scolecite, Strawberry Quartz, Tanzanite, Thunder Egg, Tremolite,

Tugtupite. *Chakra:* earth star, base

Apathy: Brookite, Bushman Red Cascade, Chinese Red Quartz, Macedonian Opal, Poppy Jasper, Zebra Stone. *Chakra:* base, sacral, dantien

Aphrodisiac: see Libido page 137

Apoptosis (cell death and regeneration): Gabbro, Granite, Klinoptilolith. *Chakra:* dantien

Appetite:

> **suppressant:** Lepidocrosite. *Chakra:* solar plexus
>
> **regulate:** Pearl Spa Dolomite. *Chakra:* sacral

Arrogance: Covellite, Diopside. *Chakra:* base and soma

Arteries: Chohua Jasper, Chrysotile, Graphic Smoky Quartz (Zebra Stone), Rainbow Moonstone

> **blocked:** Brucite, Chalcanthite. *Chakra:* heart

Arteriosclerosis: Chalcanthite, Pyrite in Magnesite

Arthritis: Aztee, Blue Euclase, Brochantite, Calcite Fairy Stone, Chalcanthite, Chalcopyrite, Chinese Red Quartz, Dianite, Nzuri Moyo, Paraiba Tourmaline, Prophecy Stone, Plancheite, Rhodozite, Shungite, Wind Fossil Agate and see Joints page 131 and Pain relief page 159

Asbestos related tumour: Actinolite, Champagne Aura Quartz, Klinoptilolith

Ascension process, assist: Nirvana Quartz, Sanda Rosa Azeztulite. *Chakra:* higher crown

Assertion: Bronzite. *Chakra:* base, sacral

Assimilation of: *Chakra:* dantien, solar plexus

> **calcium:** Bustamite, Cavansite, Hackmanite,

Unless otherwise directed, apply crystal over organ or site of symptom, place on appropriate chakra, wear as jewellery, bathe with or take as a crystal essence.

Serpentine in Obsidian, Stone of Dreams
carbohydrates: Candle Quartz
copper: Dendritic Chalcedony, Limonite
iodine: Blue Halite
iron: Bronzite, Enstatite and Diopside, Girasol, Limonite, Phantom Calcite
minerals: Kambaba Jasper, Khutnohorite, Piemontite, Tantalite
nutrients: Anthrophyllite, Candle Quartz, Coprolite, Klinoptilolith, Orchid Calcite, Phlogopite, Smoky Amethyst
oxygen: Goethite, Pyrite in Quartz, Snakeskin Pyrite, Sonora Sunrise
phosphorous: Dinosaur Bone
potassium: Bornite
protein: Phantom Calcite, Picrolite
vitamin A, B and E: Creedite
vitamin C: Orchid Calcite
vitamins: Orchid Calcite, Phlogopite, Kambaba Jasper
Asthma: Banded Agate, Catlinite (Pipestone), Dianite, Nzuri Moyo, Pyrite in Quartz, Riebekite with Sugilite and Bustamite, Shungite, Tremolite. *Chakra:* solar plexus, dantien, higher heart (or wear constantly over chest, take as crystal essence)
Astigmatism: see Eyes page 108
Astral projection/journeying: Afghanite, Nuummite,

Scolecite, Sedona Stone, Stibnite, Titanite (Sphene). Chakra: third eye, soma, crown, and see Journeying page 132 and Travel page 150

> **facilitate:** double-terminated crystals (hold or apply to soma/third eye chakra)
>
> **protection during:** Nunderite, Stibnite (hold or wear)
>
> **prevention:** Banded Agate, Faden Quartz (wear constantly at night or place by bed)

Athletes: Benitoite

Atmospheric pollutants: Elestial Quartz, Nuummite, Paraiba Tourmaline, Pyrite and Sphalerite, Quantum Quattro, Shaman Quartz, Shungite. *Chakra:* earth star

Attachments: Drusy Golden Healer, Ilmenite, Larvikite, Rainbow Mayanite, Stibnite, Smoky Amethyst, Tantalite, Tinguaite, and see Spirit release page 188

Attention deficit disorder: see ADHD page 51

Authority figures, difficulties with: Sonora Sunrise

Attitude, to change: Amethyst Spirit Quartz, Axinite, Dream Quartz, Drusy Danburite, Eclipse Stone, Fluorapatite, Heulandite, Lilac Crackle Quartz, Luxullianite, Purpurite, Satyaloka Quartz, Smoky Citrine, Stichtite, Wavellite, see page 82

Aura: Anandalite™, Beryllonite, Scolecite (hold in front of solar plexus or sweep aura)

> **align with physical body:** Ajo Blue Calcite, Anandalite, Empowerite, Larvikite, Schalenblende, Scheelite, Scolecite, Sichuan Quartz, Sillimanite,

---

Unless otherwise directed, apply crystal over organ or site of symptom, place on appropriate chakra, wear as jewellery, bathe with or take as a crystal essence.

Thompsonite (hold over head or solar plexus)

align with spiritual energy: Annabergite, Andrean Blue Opal, Celadonite, Ethiopian Opal, Prophecy Stone, Ruby Lavender Quartz, Sillimanite. *Chakra:* crown, soul star, stellar gateway

blockages, remove: Ajo Quartz, Arfvedsonite, Beryllonite, Fire and Ice Quartz, Prehnite with Epidote, Rhodozite, Serpentine in Obsidian

cleansing: Amechlorite, Anandalite, Black Kyanite, Citrine Spirit Quartz, Fire and Ice Quartz, Flint, Holly Agate, Keyiapo, Lepidocrosite, Mystic Topaz, Nuummite, Phlogopite, Pumice, Pyrite in Quartz, Pyrite and Sphalerite, Rainbow Mayanite, Rutile ('comb' aura thoroughly)

cords, remove: Amechlorite, Lemurian Aquitane Calcite, Nunderite, Nuummite with Novaculite, Rainbow Mayanite

energize: Anandalite™, Gold in Quartz, Sichuan Quartz. *Chakra:* solar plexus

energy leakage, guard against: Eudialyte, Gaspeite, Pyrite in Quartz, Quartz with Mica, Spectrolite. *Chakra:* higher heart (wear constantly)

entities, remove: Amechlorite, Drusy Golden Healer, Keyiapo, Klinoptilolith, Larvikite, Pyromorphite, Selenite Phantom, and see Entities page 106. *Chakra:* base, sacral, solar plexus, spleen, third eye

heal: Keyiapo, Piemontite, Scolecite, Sichuan Quartz,

Unless otherwise directed, apply crystal over organ or site of symptom, place on appropriate chakra, wear as jewellery, bathe with or take as a crystal essence.

Smoky Amethyst, Tugtupite

'holes'/breaks: Aegerine, Brookite, Chinese Red Quartz, Eye of the Storm, Green Ridge Quartz, Lemurian Seed, Scolecite (place over site)

implants/mental attachments, remove: Amechlorite, Chinese Red Quartz, Cryolite, Drusy Golden Healer, Holly Agate, Ilmenite, Klinoptilolith, Lemurian Aquitane Calcite, Molybdenite in Quartz, Rainbow Mayanite, Tantalite, Tinguaite. *Chakra:* third eye (place on chakra until released, then purify stone immediately)

negativity, remove: Nuummite with Novaculite, Smoky Amethyst, Spectrolite, Tantalite. *Chakra:* solar plexus.

negative patterns embedded in, dissolve: Amechlorite, Amphibole, Arfvedsonite, Bronzite, Flint, Garnet in Quartz, Glendonite, Nuummite with Novaculite, Rainbow Covellite, Rainbow Mayanite, Scheelite, Spectrolite, Tantalite ('comb' over aura)

protect: Honey Phantom Calcite, Hackmanite, Mahogany Sheen Obsidian, Master Shamanite, Nunderite, Paraiba Tourmaline, Tantalite. *Chakra:* higher heart (wear continuously)

seal: Actinolite, Andean Blue Opal, Brookite, Feather Pyrite, Galaxyite, Honey Phantom Calcite, Lorenzenite (Ramsayite), Molybdenite in Quartz, Nunderite, Pyromorphite, Smoky Amethyst,

Serpentine in Obsidian, Spectrolite, Tantalite, Thunder Egg, Valentinite and Stibnite, Xenotine

stabilize: Granite, Mtrolite, Poppy Jasper. *Chakra:* earth star

strengthen: Ajo Blue Calcite, Brookite, Ethiopian Opal, Flint, Tantalite, Thunder Egg

weakness, overcome: Brookite

Autoimmune diseases: Bastnasite, Brandenberg Amethyst, Chinese Red Quartz, Diaspore (Zultanite), Gabbro, Granite, Mookaite Jasper, Paraiba Tourmaline, Richterite, Rosophia, Shungite, Tangerose, Titanite (Sphene), Winchite. *Chakra:* dantien, higher heart

Autonomic nervous system: Alexandrite, Anglesite. *Chakra:* dantien

---

- B -

Back: Petrified Wood

    disc elasticity: Calcite Fairy Stone, Strontianite

    impacted vertebrae: Faden Quartz, Graphic Smoky Quartz (Zebra Stone), White Phantom Quartz

    lower: Bastnasite, Flint, Quantum Quattro, Mtrolite, Scheelite

    pain: Bastnasite, Blue Euclase, Cathedral Quartz, Flint, Quantum Quattro, Mtrolite, Rhodozite

Bacteria, proliferate helpful: Amechlorite

Bacterial infections: Richterite, Shungite (bathe in crystal essence or place stone over site)

Bad:

    breath: Blue Crackle Quartz

    temper, ameliorate: Neptunite, Pearl Spa Dolomite

Baggage, releasing emotional: Chrysotile in Serpentine, Eclipse Stone, Cumberlandite, Garnet in Quartz, Graphic Smoky Quartz (Zebra Stone), Mount Shasta Opal, Tangerose, Tanzine Aura Quartz, Tremolite, Tugtupite, Wind Fossil Agate, Xenotine. *Chakra:* solar plexus, heart

Balance:

    Body-mind-spirit: Actinolite, Larvikite, Merlinite

    male/female energies: Alexandrite, Amphibole Quartz, Day and Night Quartz, Khutnohorite. *Chakra:* base and sacral

    mineral content: Bird's Eye Jasper, Poppy Jasper.

Unless otherwise directed, apply crystal over organ or site of symptom, place on appropriate chakra, wear as jewellery, bathe with or take as a crystal essence.

Chakra: solar plexus and see Assimilation page 56

physical body with etheric: Ajoite, Andara Glass, Astraline, Eye of the Storm, Granite, Larvikite, Nuummite, Rutile with Hematite, Sanda Rosa Azeztulite, Mohawkite, Thompsonite

physical body with lightbody: Golden Coracalcite, Golden Healer Quartz, Prophecy Stone, Red Celestial Madagascan Quartz, Scheelite, Scolecite, Victorite

vibrational shifts: Anandalite™, Lemurian Gold Opal, Lemurian Seed

yin-yang: Amphibole, Dalmatian Stone, Day and Night Quartz, Eilat Stone, Merlinite, Morion, Poppy Jasper, Spirit Quartz, Shiva Lingam. *Chakra:* sacral, dantien (or wear continuously)

Baldness: see Hair page 117

Base chakra: see Chakras page 76

Bedsores: Shungite

Beliefs that no longer serve: Goethite. *Chakra:* past life, third eye

Belonging: Polychrome Jasper. *Chakra:* earth star, base, dantien

Beta brainwaves: see Brain page 69

Betrayal: Quantum Quattro, Smoky Rose Quartz, Tugtupite

Bigotry, overcome effects of: Tugtupite. *Chakra:* heart

Bile: Biotite, Heulandite, Kambaba Jasper

    duct blockages: Gaspeite, Poppy Jasper, Pyrite and

Sphalerite, Rhodozite, Serpentine in Obsidian

regulate excess: Rosophia

Biliousness: Green Calcite, Gaspeite. *Chakra:* solar plexus

Biomagnetic field destabilized: Anandalite and see Aura page 58. *Chakra:* dantien, solar plexus

Biorhythmic clock: Fluorapatite, Kambaba Jasper, Stromatolite. *Chakra:* dantien, higher heart or alta major (base of skull)

Bipolar disorder: Bastnasite, Brucite, Halite, Lepidocrosite, Montebrasite, Tantalite. *Chakra:* third eye

Birth: Covellite, Menalite. *Chakra:* sacral (hold or bind over abdomen)

> **birth canal, opening:** Crackled Fire Agate, Picture Jasper, Poppy Jasper
>
> **pain, lessen:** Blue Euclase, Cathedral Quartz, Menalite, Poppy Jasper, Rhodozite
>
> **pre, issues:** Voegesite

Bites, venomous: Serpentine, Stichtite (apply to site)

Bitterness: Gaspeite, Huebnerite

Bladder: Conichalcite, Libyan Gold Tektite, Prehnite with Epidote, Rosophia, Sonora Sunrise, Stromatolite. *Chakra:* dantien

Bleeding: Poppy Jasper

> **cauterize/stop:** Poppy Jasper, Purpurite (apply over site)
>
> **excessive:** Purpurite
>
> **nose:** Purpurite

Unless otherwise directed, apply crystal over organ or site of symptom, place on appropriate chakra, wear as jewellery, bathe with or take as a crystal essence.

menstrual, excessive: Eilat Stone

Bloating: Ocean Jasper, Ocean Blue Jasper

Blockages, self-imposed: Bowenite (New Jade), Brandenberg Amethyst, Elestial Quartz, Gold Siberian Quartz, Prehnite with Epidote, Rhodozite, Serpentine in Obsidian, Sichuan Quartz. *Chakra:* higher heart

Blocked feelings: Indicolite Quartz, Pyrite in Quartz, Pyrite and Sphalerite, Tanzine Aura Quartz

Blood: Agnitite™, Amechlorite, Cinnabar in Jasper, Garnet in Pyroxene, Poppy Jasper, Red Amethyst, Tugtupite. *Chakra:* heart, spleen

  brain-barrier: Brochantite

  cells: Erythrite, Pink Sunstone

  cells, red to white ratio: Bixbite

  cells, unclump: Anandalite™, Shungite

  circadian rhythm: Fluorapatite. *Chakra:* dantien, alta major (base of skull)

  circulation: Anglesite, Budd Stone (African Jade), Cinnabar in Jasper, Clinohumite, Garnet in Quartz, Green Diopside, Hilulite, Prophecy Stone, Riebekite with Sugilite and Bustamite, Roselite, Tugtupite

  cleanser: Amechlorite, Cinnabar in Jasper. *Chakra:* spleen

  clots, dissolve: Arsenopyrite, Hematoid Calcite, Plancheite

  clotting, slow: Pyrite in Magnesite

  corpuscles, red: Orange River Red Quartz

Unless otherwise directed, apply crystal over organ or site of symptom, place on appropriate chakra, wear as jewellery, bathe with or take as a crystal essence.

detox: Amechlorite, Eye of the Storm, Halite, Larvikite, Pyrite in Magnesite

disorders: Atlantasite, Benitoite, Hemimorphite, Malacholla, Rainbow Covellite, Richterite, Shungite, Smoky Quartz with Aegerine

faulty oxygenation: Hematoid Calcite, Klinoptilolith, Orange River Quartz, Quantum Quattro, Pyrite in Quartz, Snakeskin Pyrite, Sonora Sunrise, Stone of Solidarity

flow in liver: Cinnabar in Jasper, Garnet in Pyroxene, Orange River Quartz, Red Amethyst, Tugtupite

purification: Hematoid Calcite, Ussingite

red: Bixbite, Cinnabar in Jasper, Orange River Quartz, Tugtupite

supply to organs: Feather Pyrite

vessels: Blue Euclase, Hausmanite, Rutile, Scheelite, Tugtupite

Blood pressure:

equalize: Cat's Eye Quartz, Diopside, Hackmanite, Stichtite, Smoky Rose Quartz, Stichtite and Serpentine, Tanzanite, Tanzine Aura Quartz, Tugtupite, Ussingite. *Chakra:* dantien, heart

high: Cat's Eye Quartz, Eye of the Storm, Larvikite, Quantum Quattro, Reinerite, Richterite, Stichtite, Stichtite and Serpentine, Tanzine Aura Quartz, Tugtupite. *Chakra:* dantien, heart

low: Green Diopside. *Chakra:* heart

Unless otherwise directed, apply crystal over organ or site of symptom, place on appropriate chakra, wear as jewellery, bathe with or take as a crystal essence.

Blood sugar imbalances: Astraline, Chinese Chromium Quartz, Chrome Diopside, Green Shaman Quartz, Huebnerite, Maw Sit Sit, Malacholla, Mtrolite, Orange Kyanite, Owyhee Blue Opal, Pink Opal, Pink Sunstone, Serpentine in Obsidian, Shungite, Stichtite and Serpentine, Tugtupite and see Diabetes page 96 and Pancreas page 128. *Chakra*: spleen, dantien, heart

Blueprint, etheric: Anandalite, Andescine Labradorite, Astraline, Black Kyanite, Beryllonite, Brandenberg Amethyst, Ethiopian Opal, Eye of the Storm, Keyiapo, Khutnohorite, Lemurian Aquitane Calcite, Pollucite, Rhodozite, Ruby Lavender Quartz, Sanda Rosa Azeztulite, Scheelite, Seriphos Quartz, Tantalite. *Chakra:* soma

Body:

   discomfort at being in: Pearl Spa Dolomite, Quantum Quattro, Strontianite. *Chakra*: earth star, base, sacral, dantien

   fluids, balance: Azeztulite with Morganite, Bastnasite, Hackmanite, Nunderite, Scheelite, Smoky Amethyst, Trigonic Quartz. *Chakra*: earth star, base, sacral

   heat, excess: Brazilianite. *Chakra*: earth star, base, sacral issues: Azotic Topaz

   odour: Leopardskin Jasper. *Chakra*: earth star, base, sacral

   promote repair: Bixbite, Tantalite, and see Cellular

Unless otherwise directed, apply crystal over organ or site of symptom, place on appropriate chakra, wear as jewellery, bathe with or take as a crystal essence.

healing page 75. *Chakra*: earth star, base, sacral

strengthen: Blue Aragonite, Erythrite, Fiskenaesset Ruby, Poppy Jasper. *Chakra*: earth star, base, sacral, dantien

Boils: Quantum Quattro, Shungite

Bombarded by other people's thoughts: Auralite 23, Larvikite, Mohawkite, Scolecite, Tantalite. *Chakra:* third eye (or wear continuously)

Bones: Brookite, Cat's Eye Quartz, Cradle of Life, Cryolite, Feather Pyrite, Fluorapatite, Golden Coracalcite, Hausmanite, Khutnohorite, Marialite, Petrified Wood, Piemontite, Poldervaarite, Pyrite in Magnesite, Scolecite, Shell Jasper, Stone of Dreams, Strontianite, Titanite (Sphene), Wind Fossil Agate

aching: Cradle of Life

brittle: Faden Quartz, Fire and Ice Quartz, Pink Crackle Quartz, Scolecite, Trummer Jasper

broken: Axinite, Creedite, Faden Quartz, Glendonite, Graphic Smoky Quartz (Zebra Stone), Nzuri Moyo, Oligoclase

disease: Zebra Stone

disorders: Graphic Smoky Quartz, Scolecite

growth: Diaspore (Zultanite), Cavansite, Khutnohorite, Piemontite

healing: Cradle of Life, Eilat Stone

loss: Cavansite

marrow: Erythrite, Goethite

Unless otherwise directed, apply crystal over organ or site of symptom, place on appropriate chakra, wear as jewellery, bathe with or take as a crystal essence.

strengthening: Pink Crackle Quartz, Glendonite, Graphic Smoky Quartz, Scolecite

structure: Cradle of Life, Graphic Smoky Quartz, Hausmanite, Khutnohorite

Bone-marrow disorders: Cradle of Life, Goethite

Boundaries: Brazilianite, Lemurian Jade, Serpentine in Obsidian, Tantalite. *Chakra:* solar plexus (or wear continuously)

Bowels: Xenotine. *Chakra:* dantien

blockage: Ajoite with Shattuckite, Pyrite in Quartz, Pyrite and Sphalerite, Rhodozite, Rosophia

Brain: Brandenberg Amethyst, Crystal Cap Amethyst, Epidote, Nuummite, Prehnite with Epidote, Pyrite and Sphalerite, Schalenblende, Trigonic Quartz, White Heulandite, Vera Cruz Amethyst. *Chakra:* third eye, soma, crown, alta major

balance left–right hemispheres: Cumberlandite, Crystal Cap Amethyst, Eudialyte, Lilac Quartz, Rhodozite, Stromatolite, Trigonic Quartz. *Chakra:* soma

benign tumours: Scolecite

beta waves: Brandenberg Amethyst, Blue Euclase, Crystal Cap Amethyst, Spirit Quartz, Spirit Quartz, Vera Cruz Amethyst. *Chakra:* third eye, crown

blood flow, improve: Poppy Jasper, Tugtupite

chemistry: Barite, Stichtite

damage: Amphibole, Anthrophyllite, Brandenberg

Unless otherwise directed, apply crystal over organ or site of symptom, place on appropriate chakra, wear as jewellery, bathe with or take as a crystal essence.

Amethyst, Galaxyite, Herderite

degeneration: Anthrophyllite

detox: Amechlorite, Eye of the Storm, Klinoptilolith, Larvikite, Nuummite, Rainbow Covellite, Rhodozite, Richterite, Shungite, Smoky Quartz with Aegerine

disorders: Brandenberg Amethyst, Chalcopyrite, Galaxyite, Holly Agate, Khutnohorite

fatigue: Apricot Quartz, Pyrite in Quartz, Strawberry Lemurian

frequencies: Crystal Cap Amethyst, Lilac Quartz, Satyaloka and Satyamani Quartz, Vera Cruz Amethyst

function: Cryolite, Phantom Calcite, Rhodozite

left: Realgar and Orpiment

neural pathways: Anglesite, Celestobarite, Crystal Cap Amethyst, Feather Calcite, Feather Pyrite, Holly Agate, Larvikite, Phantom Calcite, Pyrite and Sphalerite, Schalenblende, Scolecite, Stichtite

right: Merkabite Calcite

stem: Blue Moonstone, Cradle of Life, Chrysotile, Chrysotile in Serpentine, Eye of the Storm, Kambaba Jasper, Schalenblende, Stromatolite

theta waves: Brandenberg Amethyst, Trigonic Quartz

tumour: Champagne Aura Quartz, Eilat Stone, Klinoptilolith, Nuummite, Ouro Verde

waves, harmonize: Blue Euclase, Brandenberg Amethyst, Spirit Quartz, Eudialyte

Breastfeeding: Menalite and see Lactation page 136

Unless otherwise directed, apply crystal over organ or site of symptom, place on appropriate chakra, wear as jewellery, bathe with or take as a crystal essence.

Breath work: Blue Aragonite, Riebekite with Sugilite and Bustamite. *Chakra:* dantien

Breathlessness: Blue Crackle Quartz, Riebekite with Sugilite and Bustamite, Tremolite. *Chakra:* dantien, solar plexus, throat

Breathing disorders: Blue Aragonite, Blue Crackle Quartz, Hanksite, Riebekite with Sugilite and Bustamite, Tremolite. *Chakra:* dantien

Bronchitis: Cat's Eye Quartz, Chalcopyrite, Dianite, Pyrite in Quartz, Richterite, Riebekite with Sugilite and Bustamite, Shungite, Tremolite. *Chakra:* higher heart

Bruises: Agrellite, Crystal Cap Amethyst, Dream Quartz, Gabbro, Purpurite, Amethyst

Brow chakra: see Third Eye, Chakras, pages 76–82

Bulimia: Dianite, Orange Kyanite, Picasso Jasper. *Chakra:* solar plexus

Bullying: Cat's Eye Quartz. *Chakra:* dantien (or keep in pocket)

Burning sensation: Lilac Quartz

Burn-out: Crackled Fire Agate, Marcasite, Poppy Jasper, Que Sera, Quantum Quattro, Strawberry Lemurian. *Chakra:* base, dantien

Burns: Amphibole, Hemimorphite, Indicolite, Klinoptilolith, Lilac Quartz (place stone in cold water and immerse burn for 20 minutes)

Unless otherwise directed, apply crystal over organ or site of symptom, place on appropriate chakra, wear as jewellery, bathe with or take as a crystal essence.

- C -

Calcification: Calcite Fairy Stone, Dream Quartz, Menalite, Petrified Wood

Calcium: see Assimilation page 56

calcium-magnesium balance: Serpentine in Obsidian. *Chakra:* heart, solar plexus

deficiency: Bustamite, Cavansite

Calluses: Pumice, Wind Fossil Agate

Calming:

emotions: Mount Shasta Opal, Oceanite, Tugtupite

fear: Arsenopyrite, Eilat Stone, Graphic Smoky Quartz (Zebra Stone), Guardian Stone, Khutnohorite, Oceanite, Scolecite, Tangerose, Thunder Egg

physical body: Jamesonite, Scolecite. *Chakra:* dantien

Cancer: Eilat Stone, Fluorapatite, Gabbro, Klinoptilolith (place over site), Malacholla, Rhodozite, Shungite (drink as Shungite water), Sonora Sunrise and see Tumours page 198

support during: Amethyst Spirit Quartz, Bixbite, Black Diopside, Brandenberg Amethyst, Cathedral Quartz, Cassiterite, Cobalto Calcite, Dendritic Chalcedony, Epidote, Eye of the Storm, Green Ridge Quartz, Hemimorphite, Icicle Calcite, Lemurian Jade, Paraiba Tourmaline, Quantum Quattro, Reinerite, Rhodozite, Sonora Sunrise, Tremolite, Winchite

Capillaries: Feather Pyrite

Unless otherwise directed, apply crystal over organ or site of symptom, place on appropriate chakra, wear as jewellery, bathe with or take as a crystal essence.

Carbohydrate assimilation: see Assimilation page 56

Carbuncle: Shungite (tape over site)

Cardiothoracic system: Purpurite and see Heart page 119

Cardiovascular system: Shungite, Tugtupite and see Heart page 119

Carpel tunnel syndrome: Frondellite (use as wrist rest)

Cataracts: Blue Chalcedony, Marialite, Scapolite, Vivianite

Catarrh: see Mucus page 149

Cartilage: Dalmatian Stone

Causes of disease:

    anxiety or fear: Candle Quartz, Dumortierite, Eilat Stone, Khutnohorite, Oceanite, Tangerose, Thunder Egg, Tremolite, Tugtupite. *Chakra:* solar plexus

    damaged immune system: Brandenberg Amethyst, Blizzard Stone, Diaspore (Zultanite), Gabbro, Lemurian Jade, Mookaite Jasper, Nzuri Moyo, Ocean Blue Jasper, Pyrite and Sphalerite, Que Sera, Quantum Quattro, Schalenblende, Shungite, Stone of Solidarity, Super 7, Tangerose, Titanite (Sphene), Winchite. *Chakra:* dantien, higher heart

    emotional exhaustion: Candle Quartz, Mount Shasta Opal, Prehnite with Epidote. *Chakra:* solar plexus

    mental stress: Candle Quartz, Eye of the Storm, Guinea Fowl Jasper, Lemurian Gold Opal, Richterite, Shungite. *Chakra:* third eye, soma

---

Unless otherwise directed, apply crystal over organ or site of symptom, place on appropriate chakra, wear as jewellery, bathe with or take as a crystal essence.

negative attitudes or emotions: Candle Quartz, Kornerupine, Pyrite in Quartz, Thunder Egg

past life: Dumortierite and see Past life healing page 162

shock, trauma or psychic attack: Apricot Quartz, Empowerite, Guardian Stone, Linerite, Mohave Turquoise, Mohawkite, Oceanite, Polychrome Jasper, Tantalite, Richterite, Ruby Lavender Quartz, Victorite

stress and tension: Basalt, Bird's Eye Jasper, Bustamite, Eye of the Storm, Marble, Richterite, Riebekite with Sugilite and Bustamite, Shungite, Tugtupite

underlying, discover: Faden Quartz, Indicolite Quartz, Pholocomite

Cauterization: Andean Blue Opal, Flint, Novaculite, Seriphos Quartz

Celibacy, reverse vow of: Anandalite™, Dragon Stone, Kundalini Quartz, Serpentine in Obsidian, Smoky Citrine

Cells:

detox: Eye of the Storm, Klinoptilolith, Larvikite, Smoky Quartz with Aegerine, Shungite

energetic balance: Lemurian Gold Opal, Rainbow Covellite, Richterite, Sanda Rosa Azeztulite, Shungite. *Chakra:* dantien

metabolism: Ammolite, Pyrite in Magnesite, Tangerine Sun Aura Quartz

production: Bixbite

repair: Bixbite, Glendonite, Rosophia
walls: Calcite Fairy Stone, Eye of the Storm, Feather Pyrite, Poppy Jasper, Titanite (Sphene). *Chakra:* dantien

Cell phones, protection against emanations: Elestial Smoky Quartz, Quantum Quattro, Shungite (tape to phone)

Cellular:
blueprint: Ajoite, Ajo Quartz, Brandenberg Amethyst, Eye of the Storm, Keyiapo, Khutnohorite, Rhodozite, Ruby Lavender Quartz, Scheelite, Seriphos Quartz. *Chakra:* higher heart, soma, alta major (base of skull)

disorders: Biotite, Eye of the Storm, Pyrite in Magnesite, Rhodozite, Shungite

detoxification: Eye of the Storm, Kambaba Jasper, Larvikite, Rainbow Covellite, Richterite, Shungite, Smoky Quartz with Aegerine, Stromatolite, Tantalite

healing: Ajo Quartz, Brandenberg Amethyst, Crystal Cap Amethyst, Elestial Quartz, Eudialyte, Eye of the Storm, Khutnohorite, Mangano Vesuvianite, Marialite, Pyrite in Magnesite, Rainbow Mayanite, Rainforest Jasper, Reinerite, Rhodozite, Rosophia, Schalenblende, Tantalite, Titanite (Sphene)

matrix: Gold in Quartz

memory: Ajo Quartz, Ajoite, Andean Blue Opal, Azotic Topaz, Brandenberg Amethyst, Bustamite,

Chrysotile, Datolite, Dumortierite, Eilat Stone, Elestial Quartz, Eye of the Storm, Heulandite, Lepidocrosite, Leopardskin Jasper, Nuummite, Rainbow Mayanite, Rhodozite, Sichuan Quartz, Smoky Quartz with Aegerine, Spirit Quartz, Valentinite and Stibnite. *Chakra:* dantien, alta major

micro level: Ruby Lavender Quartz

processes: Eye of the Storm, Feather Pyrite

regeneration: Andean Blue Opal, Elestial Quartz, Eye of the Storm, Lepidocrosite, Reinerite, Rosophia, Shungite, Tantalite

structure: Ajo Quartz, Ajoite, Bornite, Cradle of Life, Lilac Quartz, Hausmanite, Messina Quartz, Novaculite, Reinerite, Rhodozite, Shungite

swelling: Anandalite™, Gabbro

wall reprogramming: Calcite Fairy Stone, Eye of the Storm, Feather Pyrite, Poppy Jasper, Titanite (Sphene). *Chakra:* dantien

Centring: Stichtite and Serpentine

Central nervous system, depleted or disturbed: Anandalite™, Anglesite, Larvikite, Natrolite with Scolecite, Prehnite with Epidote. *Chakra:* dantien (wear continuously)

Cerebellum: Anthrophyllite, Kambaba Jasper, Stromatolite, Shungite. *Chakra:* third eye, crown

Cervix: Menalite, Calcite Fairy Stone. *Chakra:* sacral

Chakras:

Unless otherwise directed, apply crystal over organ or site of symptom, place on appropriate chakra, wear as jewellery, bathe with or take as a crystal essence.

activate all: Anandalite, Brookite, Golden Healer Quartz, Phlogopite, Rhodozite, Victorite

activate higher crown: Amphibole, Anandalite, Angels Wing Calcite, Brookite, Diaspore (Zultanite), Glendonite, Golden Healer Quartz, Lemurian Aquitane Calcite, Lepidocrosite, Merkabite Calcite™, Novaculite, Paraiba Tourmaline, Titanite (Sphene), Victorite (place above head)

activate higher heart: Ajo Blue Calcite, Macedonian Opal, Pink Lazurine, Pyroxmangite, Roselite, Ruby Lavender Quartz, Scolecite (place over thymus)

align: Anandalite, Auralite 23, Brochantite, Golden Healer Quartz, Lemurian Seed, Montebrasite, Novaculite, Rhodozite, Sillimanite

align with physical body: Anandalite, Celestial Quartz, Keyiapo, Lemurian Jade, Lemurian Seed, Morion, Prasiolite, Preseli Bluestone, Rhodozite, Sillimanite, Smoky Herkimer Diamond, Sichuan Quartz, Thompsonite

Alta Major: Afghanite, African Jade, Angelinite, Apatite, Anandalite, Andara Glass, Angels Wing Calcite, Auralite 23, Aurichalcite, Azeztulite, Blue Moonstone, Brandenberg Amethyst, Budd Stone (African Jade), Crystal Cap Amethyst, Diaspore (Zultanite), Ethiopian Opal, Eye of the Storm (Judy's Jasper), Fire and Ice Quartz, Garnet in Pyroxene, Graphic Smoky Quartz, Green Ridge Quartz, Golden

Herkimer Diamond, Golden Healer, Holly Agate, Hungarian Quartz, Petalite, Phenacite, Preseli Bluestone, Fluorapatite, Red Agate, Rainbow Covellite, Rainbow Mayanite, Red Amethyst, Rosophia (place at base of skull)

balance: Auralite 23, Black Kyanite, Golden Healer Quartz, Lemurian Seed, Sichuan Quartz

base: Bastnasite, Chinese Red Quartz, Clinohumite, Judy's Jasper, Kambaba Jasper, Keyiapo, Limonite, Poppy Jasper, Sonora Sunrise, Stromatolite (place at perineum)

blockages: Ajo Quartz, Amechlorite, Black Kyanite, Golden Healer Quartz, Lemurian Seed, Picrolite, Prehnite with Epidote, Pyrite and Sphalerite, Rhodozite, Sanda Rosa Azeztulite

cleanse: Anandalite, Enstatite and Diopside, Flint, Golden Healer Quartz, Graphic Smoky Quartz (Zebra Stone), Orange Kyanite, Novaculite, Nuummite, Rainbow Mayanite, Rhodozaz, Rhodozite,

connect higher: Astraline, Rosophia, Rhodozaz, Titanite (Sphene)

crown: Afghanite, Amphibole Quartz, Arfvedsonite, Novaculite, Rosophia, Satyamani and Satyaloka Quartz, Titanite (Sphene) (place on top of head)

dantien: Empowerite, Eye of the Storm, Golden Herkimer, Hematoid Calcite, Kambaba Jasper, Peanut Wood, Polychrome Jasper, Poppy Jasper, Red

Unless otherwise directed, apply crystal over organ or site of symptom, place on appropriate chakra, wear as jewellery, bathe with or take as a crystal essence.

Amethyst, Rhodozite, Rose or Ruby Aura Quartz, Rosophia, Stromatolite

Earth Star: Agnitite™, Celestobarite, Flint, Graphic Smoky Quartz, Golden Herkimer, Lemurian Jade, Limonite, Proustite, Red Amethyst, Rhodozite, Rosophia, Smoky Elestial Quartz, Thunder Egg (place below feet)

ground energies through: Aztee, Champagne Aura Quartz, Empowerite, Keyiapo, Mohawkite, Peanut Wood, Polychrome Jasper, Red Amethyst, Rhodozite, Schalenblende, Serpentine in Obsidian, Stromatolite, Thunder Egg. *Chakra:* earth star

energy leakage, prevent: Eudialyte, Gaspeite, Pyrite in Quartz, Tantalite, Thunder Egg. *Chakra:* dantien, spleen, solar plexus

entities, release from: Eilat Stone, Flint, Holly Agate, Keyiapo, Klinoptilolith, Larvikite, Lemurian Seed, Novaculite, Pyromorphite, Stibnite, and see Entity release page 106

heart: Cobalto Calcite, Eudialyte, Gaia Stone, Green Siberian Quartz, Lilac Quartz, Pyroxmangite, Rhodozaz, Roselite, Rosophia, Ruby Lavender Quartz, Tugtupite (place over heart)

heart seed: Ajo Blue Calcite, Brandenberg Amethyst, Danburite, Lemurian Calcite, Lilac Quartz, Lilac Quartz, Macedonian Opal, Mangano Calcite, Pyroxmangite, Rhodozaz, Roselite, Rosophia, Ruby

Unless otherwise directed, apply crystal over organ or site of symptom, place on appropriate chakra, wear as jewellery, bathe with or take as a crystal essence.

Lavender Quartz, Scolecite, Tugtupite (place at base of breastbone)

higher heart/thymus: Ajo Blue Calcite, Dream Quartz, Lazurine, Lilac Quartz, Macedonian Opal, Pink Petalite, Quantum Quattro, Pyroxmangite, Rhodozaz, Roselite, Rose Quartz Elestial, Rosophia, Ruby Lavender Quartz™, Tugtupite (place over thymus)

holes, repair: Anandalite, Barite, Black Kyanite, Lemurian Seed, Novaculite, Rainbow Mayanite

integrate higher: Montebrasite, Ruby Lavender Quartz™, Titanite (Sphene)

mental influences, detach: Flint, Novaculite, Nuummite, Rainbow Mayanite,

palm: Spangolite. *Chakra:* throat, third eye, soma, crown

past life: use appropriate crystals from Past life healing section (place behind ears)

negative karma, disturbances from: Elestial Quartz, Violane, Wind Fossil Agate

protect: Eilat Stone, Mohawkite, Tantalite, Richterite, Thunder Egg

remove blockages: Green Ridge Quartz, Lemurian Seed, Prehnite with Epidote, Pyrite and Sphalerite, Rainbow Mayanite, Rhodozite, Serpentine in Obsidian. *Chakra:* dantien

revitalize: Anandalite, Malacholla. *Chakra:* dantien

sacral/navel: Amphibole, Bastnasite, Chinese Red

Quartz, Clinohumite, Keyiapo, Limonite, Orange Kyanite (place below navel)

solar plexus: Citrine Herkimer, Golden Azeztulite, Golden Coracalcite, Golden Danburite, Golden Enhydro, Golden Healer, Green Ridge Quartz, Rhodozite, Tangerine Aura Quartz, Tangerine Dream Lemurian (place above navel)

soma: Afghanite, Amechlorite, Angelinite, Angels Wing Calcite, Astraline, Brandenberg Amethyst, Diaspore (Zultanite), Faden Quartz, Holly Agate, Merkabite Calcite, Nuummite, Preseli Bluestone, Stellar Beam Calcite

Soul Star: Afghanite, Ajoite, Amethyst Elestial, Anandalite™, Angelinite, Angels Wing Calcite, Astraline, Azeztulite, Brandenberg Amethyst, Diaspore (Zultanite), Golden Himalayan Azeztulite, Green Ridge Quartz, Holly Agate, Merkabite Calcite, Nirvana Quartz, Novaculite, Phenacite in Feldspar, Rosophia, Selenite, Satyaloka Quartz, Satyamani Quartz, Selenite, Stellar Beam Calcite, Titanite (Sphene), White Elestial (place midway on hairline)

Spleen: Gaspeite, Orange River Quartz, Prasiolite (place under left arm)

Stellar gateway: Afghanite, Amethyst Elestial, Amphibole, Anandalite™, Angelinite, Angels Wing Calcite, Astraline, Azeztulite, Brandenberg Amethyst, Diaspore (Zultanite), Fire and Ice, Golden Himalayan

Unless otherwise directed, apply crystal over organ or site of symptom, place on appropriate chakra, wear as jewellery, bathe with or take as a crystal essence.

Azeztulite, Golden Selenite, Ice Quartz, Green Ridge Quartz, Holly Agate, Merkabite Calcite, Nirvana Quartz, Novaculite, Phenacite, Stellar Beam Calcite, Titanite (Sphene), Trigonic Quartz, White Elestial Quartz (place above head)

stimulate or sedate as necessary: Poppy Jasper. *Chakra:* dantien

third eye: Afghanite, Amechlorite, Ammolite, Axinite, Black Moonstone, Blue Selenite, Bytownite, Cacoxenite, Cavansite, Glaucophane, Golden Himalayan Azeztulite, Herderite, Holly Agate, Lavender-purple Opal, Lazulite, Libyan Gold Tektite, Rhomboid Selenite, Serpentine in Obsidian, Spectrolite, Tangerine Aura Quartz (place above and between eyebrows)

throat: Astraline, Blue Quartz, Chalcanthite, Glaucophane, Green Ridge Quartz, Indicolite Quartz, Paraiba Tourmaline (place over throat)

Change:

assimilating: Actinolite, Basalt, Bismuth, Blue Euclase, Brandenberg Amethyst, Clevelandite, Conichalcite, Frondellite, Green Ridge Quartz, Luxullianite, Nunderite, Nuummite, Shift Crystal, Tangerose. *Chakra:* heart, higher heart

facilitating: Eudialyte, Ethiopian Opal, Fluorapatite, Golden Danburite, Heulandite, Luxullianite, Merlinite, Phenacite in Red Feldspar, Quantum

---

Unless otherwise directed, apply crystal over organ or site of symptom, place on appropriate chakra, wear as jewellery, bathe with or take as a crystal essence.

Quattro, Scapolite, Shaman Quartz, Snakeskin Pyrite, Tangerine Dream Lemurian. *Chakra:* heart

ground: Aztee, Basalt, Champagne Aura Quartz, Empowerite, Lemurian Jade, Libyan Gold Tektite, Mohawkite, Nunderite, Peanut Wood, Polychrome Jasper, Preseli Bluestone, Schalenblende, Serpentine in Obsidian. *Chakra:* earth star, dantien

metaphysical: Novaculite

of life: Menalite and see Menopause page 144

psychological: Annabergite, Elestial Quartz, Lilac Crackle Quartz

riding out: Datolite, Flint, Gabbro, Huebnerite, Luxullianite, Kakortokite, Montebrasite, Mtrolite, Nunderite, Ocean Jasper, Preseli Bluestone

vibrational: Anandalite™, Bismuth, Candle Quartz, Ethiopian Opal, Lemurian Gold Opal, Sanda Rosa Azeztulite, Tangerose, Tugtupite with Nuummite

Chemical pollution: Shungite, Smoky Elestial Quartz, Tantalite

Chemotherapy support: Agrellite, Eye of the Storm, Klinoptilolith, Shungite, Tremolite, Winchite

Chest: Botswana Agate. *Chakra:* dantien heart

constriction: Banded Agate, Tanzanite

pains: Blue Euclase, Eilat Stone, Quantum Quattro, Rhodozite

Chickenpox: Dalmatian Stone

Childbirth: see Birth page 64

Unless otherwise directed, apply crystal over organ or site of symptom, place on appropriate chakra, wear as jewellery, bathe with or take as a crystal essence.

Childhood, difficult: Cassiterite, Fenster Quartz, Red Phantom Quartz, Shiva Lingam, Tugtupite, Tugtupite with Nuummite, Voegesite, Youngite. *Chakra:* heart, solar plexus

Children:

> **Confidence:** Cat's Eye Quartz, Empowerite, Strontianite, Tremolite (keep in pocket)
>
> **inappropriate behaviour:** Atlantasite, Stichtite (keep in pocket)

Chills: Novaculite, Poppy Jasper, Pyrite in Magnesite

Choices: Chalcanthite, Porphyrite

Cholera: Shungite

Cholesterol, high: Andescine Labradorite, Greenlandite, Pyrite in Magnesite, Reinerite

Chromosome damage: Brandenberg Amethyst. *Chakra:* dantien, alta major

Chronic:

> **disease:** Apricot Quartz, Bismuth, Lemurian Jade, Petrified Wood, Witches Finger. *Chakra:* dantien
>
> **conditions:** Apricot Quartz, Bismuth, Diopside
>
> **exhaustion:** Apricot Quartz, Bismuth, Bronzite, Cinnabar in Jasper, Poppy Jasper, Prehnite with Epidote, Trummer Jasper. *Chakra:* dantien, higher heart
>
> **fatigue syndrome:** Adamite, Apricot Quartz, Barite, Chrysotile in Serpentine, Petrified Wood, Pyrite in Quartz, Shungite, Trummer Jasper. *Chakra:* dantien

---

Unless otherwise directed, apply crystal over organ or site of symptom, place on appropriate chakra, wear as jewellery, bathe with or take as a crystal essence.

illness: Golden Danburite, Petrified Wood, Poppy Jasper, Que Sera, Shungite, Trummer Jasper. *Chakra:* earth star, solar plexus, higher heart

Chronic sore throat: Shungite. *Chakra:* throat (or gargle with essence)

Circadian rhythm: Fluorapatite. *Chakra:* dantien, alta major

Circular breathing: Ocean Jasper. *Chakra:* dantien

Circulation: Alabaster, Anglesite, Brazilianite, Brookite, Budd Stone (African Jade), Bustamite, Clinohumite, Fiskenaesset Ruby, Garnet in Quartz, Green Diopside, Molybdenite, Morion, Ocean Jasper, Ouro Verde, Pyroxmangite, Riebekite with Sugilite and Bustamite, Rosophia, Trigonic Quartz. *Chakra:* dantien, heart

> **fortifying:** Blue Herkimer with Boulangerite, Tanzine Aura Quartz
>
> **poor:** Merlinite
>
> **peripheral:** Dianite, Ouro Verde, Spangolite

Cirrhosis: Gaspeite

Clarity, promote: Adamite, Ammolite, Blue Moonstone, Blue Quartz, Chinese Chromium Quartz, Chinese Red Quartz, Datolite, Dumortierite, Green Ridge Quartz, Holly Agate, Judy's Jasper, Lemurian Seed, Leopardskin Jasper, Limonite, Marcasite, Morion, Pearl Spa Dolomite, Purpurite, Rainforest Jasper, Scapolite, Seriphos Quartz, Silver Leaf Jasper, Realgar and Orpiment, Smoky Candle Quartz, Super 7, Tangerine Sun Aura Quartz, Tugtupite.

Unless otherwise directed, apply crystal over organ or site of symptom, place on appropriate chakra, wear as jewellery, bathe with or take as a crystal essence.

Chakra: third eye, alta major, crown

Claustrophobia: Oceanite. *Chakra:* solar plexus

Cleansing:

    aura: see Aura page 58

    emotions: see Emotions page 101

    mind: see Mind page 147

    physical body: see Physical body page 167

Clumsiness: Black Moonstone (keep in pocket)

Codependency: Bytownite, Dumortierite, Fenster Quartz, Sichuan Quartz, Vera Cruz Amethyst. *Chakra:* base, dantien

Cognitive disorders: Crystal Cap Amethyst and see Mind etc page 147. *Chakra:* alta major

Colonic irrigation: Pumice

Cold sore: Stibnite

Coldness: Barite. *Chakra:* heart

Colds: Shungite water (drink 2 litres daily), Cathedral Quartz, Galaxyite, Honey Opal, Macedonian Opal, Quantum Quattro, Que Sera, Ocean Jasper, Rainforest Jasper. *Chakra:* higher heart

Colic: Dumortierite. *Chakra:* dantien

Colon: Black Moonstone. *Chakra:* sacral

Compassion for oneself and others: Ajoite, Brandenberg Amethyst, Cobalto Calcite, Erythrite, Gaia Stone, Goethite, Green Diopside, Green Ridge Quartz, Greenlandite, Mangano Vesuvianite, Paraiba Tourmaline, Shaman Quartz, Smoky Cathedral Quartz, Starseed

Unless otherwise directed, apply crystal over organ or site of symptom, place on appropriate chakra, wear as jewellery, bathe with or take as a crystal essence.

Quartz, Tangerose, Tanzanite, Tugtupite. *Chakra:* heart seed

Complexion: Snakeskin Agate

Compulsions, overcome: Dumortierite, Fenster Quartz. *Chakra:* base

Computer stress: Eye of the Storm, Lepidolite, Shungite. *Chakra:* higher heart

Concentration, improve: Datolite, Herderite, Schalenblende. *Chakra:* third eye

Conception: Menalite. *Chakra:* base and sacral

Concern, alleviate excess: Quantum Quattro. *Chakra:* heart

Codependency: Ice Quartz, Sichuan Quartz, Vera Cruz Amethyst

Concussion: Brandenberg Amethyst

Condescension: Heulandite

Confidence: Dumortierite, Candle Quartz, Erythrite, Eudialyte, Kakortokite, Lazulite, Morion, Prasiolite, Purpurite, Strontianite. *Chakra:* base, dantien

Conflict resolution: Champagne Aura Quartz, Fluorapatite, Trigonic Quartz

Confusion, disperse: Blue Scapolite, Celestial Quartz, Crystal Cap Amethyst, Elestial Quartz, Gabbro, Hematoid Calcite, Lepidocrosite, Limonite, Kakortokite, Owyhee Blue Opal, Paraiba Tourmaline. *Chakra:* between third eye and soma

Conjunctivitis: Vivianite

Unless otherwise directed, apply crystal over organ or site of symptom, place on appropriate chakra, wear as jewellery, bathe with or take as a crystal essence.

Connective tissue: Desert Rose, Golden Coracalcite, Greenlandite, Klinoptilolith, Kornerupine, Piemontite, Tanzanite

Constipation: Ajoite with Shattuckite, Bastnasite, Cat's Eye Quartz. *Chakra:* sacral, dantien

Conscious dreaming: Bowenite (New Jade), Chinese Writing Stone, Lemurian Seed, Owyhee Blue Opal

Contraindications and cautions:

   bipolar: avoid Rainbow Mayanite, Red Bushman Quartz, Trigonic Quartz

   Bluestone: do not place in bedroom overnight

   catharsis, may induce: Barite, Epidote, Hypersthene, Smoky Spirit Quartz, Tugtupite (replace with Quantum Quattro)

   delicate/sensitive people, may overstimulate: Rainbow Moonstone, Red Bushman Quartz, Scolecite, Tanzanite, Tremolite

   depressed: avoid Granite

   dizziness, may cause: Preseli Bluestone (change direction)

   during full moon: Blue or Rainbow Moonstone

   epilepsy: Ziron, Dumortierite, Goethite

   giddiness, remove if causes: Banded Agate

   heart palpitations, if causes remove: Eilat Stone, Malachite

   headache and nausea, if causes remove: Hanksite (then place Smoky Quartz on earth star)

Unless otherwise directed, apply crystal over organ or site of symptom, place on appropriate chakra, wear as jewellery, bathe with or take as a crystal essence.

hysteria: Red Bushman Quartz

illusion, may induce: Blue or Rainbow Moonstone

insomnia: do not wear Herkimer Diamond earrings or place on third eye

misuse of power: Hanksite accelerates

negative emotions and unpleasant truths brought to light fast: Epidote, Herkimer Diamond, Nuummite

negative energy heightened if worn constantly: Epidote, Hypersthene

night terrors: Past life crystals may invoke (see page 160)

pacemakers: Zircon can cause dizziness

psychiatric conditions, paranoia or schizophrenia: Do not use crystals unless under the supervision of a qualified crystal healer

psychic attack: Bronzite may exacerbate and perpetuate

radioactive: Very dark Smoky Quartz, Uranophane

sensitive people: Tanzanite may overstimulate psychic abilities as may Rainbow or Blue Moonstone (use black or pink Moonstone instead)

selfish gain: Hanksite brings consequences forward

Tanzanite/Blue Moonstone/Rainbow Moonstone: may create uncontrolled psychic experiences or mental overload or unwanted telepathy

toehold in incarnation: avoid Gabbro with Moonstone, Llanite (Llanoite), Polychrome Jasper.

Unless otherwise directed, apply crystal over organ or site of symptom, place on appropriate chakra, wear as jewellery, bathe with or take as a crystal essence.

Chakra: earth star and soma

toxic minerals, may contain traces of (use polished stone, make crystal essence by indirect method, wash hands after handling):

Actinolite, Adamite, Andaluscite, Ajoite, Alexandrite, Almandine Garnet, Amazonite, Aquamarine, Aragonite, Arsenopyrite, Atacamite, Aurichalcite, Axinite, Azurite, Beryl, Beryllium, Biotite (ferrous), Bixbite, Black Tourmaline, Boji-stones, Bornite, Brazilianite, Brochantite, Bumble Bee Jasper, Cavansite, Cassiterite, Celestite, Cerussite, Cervanite, Chalcanthite, Chalcopyrite (Peacock Ore), Crocoite, Cryolite, Chrysoberyl, Chrysocolla, Chrysotile, Cinnabar, Conichalcite, Copper, Covellite, Cuprite, Diopside, Dioptase, Dumortierite, Emerald, Epidote, Garnet, Gem Silica, Galena, Garnierite (Falcondoite), Goshenite, Heliodor, Hessonite Garnet, Hiddenite, Jadeite, Jamesonite, Iolite, Kinoite, Klinoptilolith, Kunzite, Kyanite, Lapis Lazuli, Lazurite, Labradorite, Lepidolite, Magnetite, Malachite, Malacholla, Marcasite, Messina Quartz, Mohawkite, Moldavite, Moonstone, Moqui Balls, Morganite, Orpiment, Pargasite, Piemontite, Pietersite, Plancheite, Prehnite, Psilomelane, Pyrite, Pyromorphite, Quantum Quattro, Que Sera, Realgar, Realgar and Orpiment, Reinerite, Rhodolite Garnet, Ruby, Sapphire, Serpentine, Spessartine Garnet, Smithsonite, Sodalite, Spinel,

Spodumene, Staurolite, Stibnite, Stilbite, Sugilite, Sulphur, Sunstone, Tanzanite, Tiffany Stone, Tiger's Eye, Topaz, Torbenite, Tourmaline, Tremolite, Turquoise, Uvarovite Garnet, Uranophane, Valentinite, Vanadinite, Variscite, Vivianite, Vesuvianite, Wavellite, Wulfenite, Zircon, Zoisite

uncontrolled psychic abilities: avoid Herkimer Diamond on third eye or at ears, also Tanzanite, Rainbow or Blue Moonstone

Control freak: Chrysotile, Ice Quartz, Lazulite, Lemurian Aquitane Calcite, Spider Web Obsidian. *Chakra:* dantien

Convalescence: Bixbite, Brandenberg Amethyst, Chohua Jasper, Empowerite, Epidote, Macedonian Opal, Quantum Quattro, Que Sera, Nzuri Moyo, Stichtite, Victorite (wear constantly)

Convulsions: see Epilepsy page 107

Core:

beliefs: Anthrophyllite, Gabbro, Mohawkite, Tantalite

being: Scolecite, Stichtite and Serpentine

energy: Erythrite, Lemurian Jade, Menalite, Poppy Jasper, Silver Leaf, Jasper, Smoky Rose Quartz, Trummer Jasper. *Chakra:* dantien

stability: Crinoidal Limestone, Polychrome Jasper, Terraluminite

Corpuscles, red: see Blood page 65

Unless otherwise directed, apply crystal over organ or site of symptom, place on appropriate chakra, wear as jewellery, bathe with or take as a crystal essence.

Coughs: Chrysotile, Quantum Quattro, Que Sera, Shungite. *Chakra:* higher heart

Courage: Bixbite, Orange River Quartz, Ruby in Albite, Youngite. *Chakra:* base, sacral, heart

Cramp: Blue Euclase, Cat's Eye Quartz, Bronzite, Dumortierite, Orange Moss Agate, Pyrite in Magnesite, Serpentine in Obsidian, Smoky Amethyst

> **intestinal:** Gaspeite, Honey Calcite, Pyrite in Magnesite, Scolecite
>
> **legs:** Smoky Amethyst, Pyrite in Magnesite
>
> **muscles:** Blue Euclase, Nzuri Moyo, Zircon, Blue or White Aragonite, Pyrite in Magnesite, Strontianite
>
> **release:** Pyrite in Magnesite
>
> **stomach:** Pyrite in Magnesite
>
> **vascular:** Pyrite in Magnesite

Cranium: Ammolite

Cravings: Crackled Fire Agate, Stichtite, Tantalite. *Chakra:* dantien, solar plexus

Creative solutions: Eilat Stone. *Chakra:* dantien

Creativity, improve: Amethyst Herkimer, Bixbite, Blue Quartz, Bushman Quartz, Covellite, Eilat Stone, Girasol, Greenlandite, Icicle Calcite, Quantum Quattro, Rainforest Jasper, Septarian, Seriphos Quartz, Tangerine Sun Aura Quartz. *Chakra:* sacral, dantien.

Crohn's disease: Cryolite. *Chakra:* dantien

Crown chakra: see Chakras page 76

'Cure-all': Eye of the Storm, Golden Healer Quartz,

Unless otherwise directed, apply crystal over organ or site of symptom, place on appropriate chakra, wear as jewellery, bathe with or take as a crystal essence.

Poppy Jasper, Quantum Quattro, Que Sera, Shungite. *Chakra:* dantien, higher heart, third eye (or wear continuously)

Curses:

> **removing:** Flint, Nuummite, Purpurite, Quantum Quattro, Stibnite. *Chakra:* heart, solar plexus, third eye
> **turn back:** Bronzite (use with caution), Master Shamanite, Mohawkite, Richterite, Tantalite. *Chakra:* throat

Cyst: Faden Quartz, Klinoptilolith, Ocean Jasper, Seriphos Quartz, Thompsonite, Wind Fossil Agate

Unless otherwise directed, apply crystal over organ or site of symptom, place on appropriate chakra, wear as jewellery, bathe with or take as a crystal essence.

- D -

Damp, susceptibility to: Rainforest Jasper

Dancers: Benitoite

Dark moods, ameliorate: Tantalite, Vera Cruz Amethyst. *Chakra:* solar plexus, third eye

Deafness: see Hearing disorders page 118

Death/dying:

    assist transition: Arfvedsonite, Crocoite, Smoky Herkimer, Smoky Herkimer, Smoky Spirit Quartz. *Chakra:* higher crown (place by bed or hold)

    coming to terms with: Lemurian Jade, Menalite, Smoky Lemurian

Decision making/overcome indecision: Bytownite, Covellite, Cryolite, Eye of the Storm, Yellow Scapolite. *Chakra:* dantien

Debilitating conditions: Brookite. *Chakra:* base

Deeply troubled: Dianite

Defensive walls, dismantle: Calcite Fairy Stone

Degenerative disease: Ammolite, Budd Stone (African Jade), Holly Agate, Nuummite, Scolecite with Natrolite, Stichtite. *Chakra:* dantien, higher heart

Dehydration: Annabergite, Epidote, Limonite, Scheelite

Delusions: see also Illusions page 124

    guard against: Red Amethyst

    remove: Kinoite, Neptunite. *Chakra:* third eye

Dementia: Anthrophyllite, Atlantasite, Holly Agate,

Unless otherwise directed, apply crystal over organ or site of symptom, place on appropriate chakra, wear as jewellery, bathe with or take as a crystal essence.

Stichtite, Stichtite and Serpentine. *Chakra:* third eye, alta major

Denial: Tremolite. *Chakra:* heart

Dental pain or problems: Blue Euclase, Cathedral Quartz, Eilat Stone, Rhodozite

Depression: Ajo Blue Calcite, Clinohumite, Dianite, Eisenkiesel, Eudialyte, Flint, Macedonian Opal, Maw Sit Sit, Montebrasite, Orange Kyanite, Pink Sunstone, Porphyrite (Chinese Letter Stone), Rainbow Goethite, Sillimanite, Spider Web Obsidian, Tugtupite. *Chakra:* solar plexus (wear continuously)

Depressive psychosis: Tugtupite. *Chakra:* higher heart (wear continuously, treat under the supervision of a qualified crystal healer)

Dermatitis: Snakeskin Agate, Wavellite

Despair: Novaculite, Pyrite in Quartz, Vera Cruz Amethyst. *Chakra:* heart (wear continuously)

Despondency: Purpurite. *Chakra:* heart

Determination: Picture Jasper

Detoxification:

body: Amechlorite, Banded Agate, Barite, Conichalcite, Coprolite, Diaspore (Zultanite), Eye of the Storm, Golden Danburite, Halite, Hanksite, Hypersthene, Jamesonite, Larvikite, Pumice, Rainbow Covellite, Richterite, Shungite, Smoky Quartz with Aegerine. *Chakra:* solar plexus, earth star, base

Unless otherwise directed, apply crystal over organ or site of symptom, place on appropriate chakra, wear as jewellery, bathe with or take as a crystal essence.

emotions: Golden Danburite, Spirit Quartz. *Chakra:* solar plexus

etheric: Astraline, Brandenberg Amethyst, Ethiopian Opal, Eye of the Storm, Lemurian Aquitane Calcite, Seriphos Quartz, Spirit Quartz, Tantalite. *Chakra:* third eye

mind: Auralite 23, Thunder Egg. *Chakra:* third eye

spiritual: Eye of the Storm, Golden Danburite, Spirit Quartz. *Chakra:* crown

Digestion: Coprolite, Golden Selenite, Limonite, Steatite. *Chakra:* dantien

Disconnection from earth: Lemurian Jade, Libyan Gold Tektite, Strontianite. *Chakra:* dantien, soma

Discontent: Covellite

Disorganisation: Blue Quartz

Diabetes: Angels Wing Calcite, Atlantasite, Bastnasite, Bowenite (New Jade), Chinese Chromium Quartz, Datolite, Pink Opal, Schalenblende, Shungite, Stichtite and Serpentine, Tugtupite, and see Blood sugar page 67 and Pancreas page 159. *Chakra:* dantien, spleen

Diagnosis, assist: Blue Lemurian Seed

Diarrhoea: Bastnasite, Dumortierite, Pyrophyllite

loose green stools, especially in children: Bastnasite

Digestion: Amblygonite, Covellite, Leopardskin Jasper, Limonite, Morion, Mystic Topaz, Ocean Jasper. *Chakra:* dantien, solar plexus

Dis-ease due to stress: Amechlorite, Basalt, Bird's Eye

Jasper, Eye of the Storm, Galaxyite, Lemurian Gold Opal, Macedonian Opal, Marble, Richterite, Riebekite with Sugilite and Bustamite, Shungite, Tugtupite and see Stress page 190

Digestive:

    organs, strengthen: Bustamite, Crackled Fire Agate, Empowerite, Kambaba Jasper, Montebrasite, Pyrite in Quartz, Serpentine in Obsidian, Snakeskin Pyrite. *Chakra:* dantien, solar plexus

    tract: Anthrophyllite, Cat's Eye Quartz, Crackled Fire Agate, Serpentine in Obsidian

        calm: Bustamite, Cat's Eye Quartz

        detox: Eye of the Storm, Klinoptilolith, Larvikite, Rainbow Covellite, Richterite, Smoky Quartz with Aegerine

        stimulate: Crackled Fire Agate

        strengthen: Crackled Fire Agate, Serpentine in Obsidian

Discs, loss of elasticity: Calcite Fairy Stone, Strontianite

Disease, infectious: Chalcopyrite, Fiskenaesset Ruby, Shungite

Distress: Eye of the Storm, Lemurian Gold Opal, Owyhee Blue Opal, Tugtupite. *Chakra:* heart

Diuretic: Halite

Dizziness: Richterite, *Chakra:* dantien, crown

DNA: Eye of the Storm, *Chakra:* dantien, higher heart

    12 strand: Eye of the Storm, Leopardskin Jasper,

Quantum Quattro, Petrified Wood

ancestral: see page 54

degeneration, reverse: Cavansite, Eye of the Storm, Petrified Wood, Pyrite in Quartz, Snakeskin Pyrite

mitochondrial: Calcite Fairy Stone, Eye of the Storm, Feather Pyrite, Poppy Jasper, Titanite (Sphene). *Chakra:* dantien

repair: Brandenberg Amethyst, Eye of the Storm, Snakeskin Pyrite

Drama Queen: Creedite. *Chakra:* dantien

Dreams:

control lucid: Chinese Writing Stone, Diaspore, Drusy Golden Healer, Scolecite, Shaman Quartz

insightful: Bowenite (New Jade), Chinese Writing Stone, Owyhee Blue Opal, Rosophia

recall: Scolecite, Strawberry Quartz

work: Andaluscite, Owyhee Blue Opal, Vivianite

Dropsy: Diopside, Chohua Jasper, Prehnite with Epidote (place over kidneys)

Ducts: Gaspeite

Dysentery: Shungite

Dysfunction: Alunite, Garnet in Quartz

Dysfunctional patterns, dissolve: Alunite, Arfvedsonite, Celadonite, Dumortierite, Fenster Quartz, Garnet in Quartz, Glendonite, Rainbow Covellite, Scheelite, Stellar Beam Calcite, Spider Web Obsidian

Dyslexia: Scapolite. *Chakra:* third eye, alta major

Unless otherwise directed, apply crystal over organ or site of symptom, place on appropriate chakra, wear as jewellery, bathe with or take as a crystal essence.

Dysmorphia: Dianite
Dyspraxia: Black Moonstone. *Chakra:* third eye

Unless otherwise directed, apply crystal over organ or site of symptom, place on appropriate chakra, wear as jewellery, bathe with or take as a crystal essence.

- E -

Ears: Covellite, Eclipse Stone, Goethite, Mystic Topaz, Peanut Wood and see Hearing page 118

> **deafness:** Peanut wood
>
> **inner:** Ammolite
>
> **pain in when flying:** Ammolite, Blue Euclase, Pink Crackle Quartz, Rhodozite (hold to or behind ear)

Earth healing: Ammolite, Black Diopside, Bustamite, Cacoxenite, Celestial Quartz, Champagne Aura Quartz, Desert Rose, Dragon Stone, Granite, Greenlandite, Lemurian Jade, Mohawkite, Monazite, Rhodozite, Scolecite, Seriphos Quartz, Smoky Brandenberg Amethyst, Smoky Elestial, Specular Hematite, Stromatolite, Super 7, Tantalite, Thunder Egg, Torbernite, Witches Finger, Z-stone. *Chakra:* earth star

> **draw off negative energies:** Smoky Elestial Quartz, Tantalite and see Electromagnetic pollution page 101

Earth Star chakra: see Chakras page 76

Eating disorders: Azeztulite with Morganite, Azotic Topaz, Cassiterite, Fenster Quartz, Quartz with Lepidolite, Orange Kyanite, Picasso Jasper, Sichuan Quartz, Stichtite. *Chakra:* dantien

Eczema: Ocean Jasper, Snakeskin Agate (bathe with alcohol-free crystal essence or place in bath)

EFT: Scheelite

Egotism: Bixbite, Hematoid Calcite, Lepidocrosite,

Unless otherwise directed, apply crystal over organ or site of symptom, place on appropriate chakra, wear as jewellery, bathe with or take as a crystal essence.

Rathbunite™, Red Amethyst. *Chakra:* base, dantien

Electrical systems: Amblygonite, Cavansite, Montebrasite, Pollucite, Shiva Lingam

Electromagnetic:

field, regulate personal: Black Moonstone, Champagne Aura Quartz, Fluorapatite

pollution: Ajoite with Shattuckite, Andara Glass, Black Moonstone, Blizzard Stone, Champagne Aura Quartz, Gabbro, Hackmanite, Klinoptilolith, Morion, Poppy Jasper, Que Sera, Red Amethyst, Shungite, Smoky Elestial Quartz, Smoky Herkimer, Tantalite, Thunder Egg. (Place stones on electrical equipment or around four corners of the house.) *Chakra:* earth star

Elimination: Molybdenite, Quantum Quattro, Steatite. *Chakra:* base, dantien

Emotional/emotions: *Chakra:* solar plexus, heart

abuse: Azeztulite with Morganite, Cobalto Calcite, Eilat Stone, Lazurine, Pink Crackle Quartz, Proustite, Tugtupite. *Chakra:* sacral, heart

alienation: Cassiterite

angst: Hemimorphite

attachment: Brandenberg Amethyst, Drusy Golden Healer, Hemimorphite, Pink Crackle Quartz, Rainbow Mayanite, Tinguaite

autonomy: Faden Quartz. *Chakra:* dantien

baggage: Ajoite, Golden Healer Quartz, Rose Elestial Quartz, Tangerose. *Chakra:* solar plexus

---

Unless otherwise directed, apply crystal over organ or site of symptom, place on appropriate chakra, wear as jewellery, bathe with or take as a crystal essence.

balance: Amblygonite, Dalmatian Stone, Eilat Stone

black hole: Ajoite, Cobalto Calcite, Quantum Quattro. *Chakra:* higher heart

blackmail: Tugtupite. *Chakra:* solar plexus

blockages: Aegirine, Botswana Agate, Bowenite (New Jade), Clinohumite, Cobalto Calcite, Eilat Stone, Green Ridge Quartz, Prehnite with Epidote, Pyrite and Sphalerite, Quantum Quattro, Rainbow Mayanite, Rhodozite, Tangerose, Tanzine Aura Quartz. *Chakra:* solar plexus

blockages from past lives: Aegirine, Datolite, Dumortierite, Graphic Smoky Quartz (Zebra Stone), Prehnite with Epidote, Pyrite and Sphalerite, Quantum Quattro, Rhodozite, Rose Elestial Quartz, Serpentine in Obsidian, and see Past life healing page 160. *Chakra:* past life

bond in relationships, heal weak: Dumortierite, Ice Quartz, Quantum Quattro, Rutile, Strawberry Quartz, Vivianite. *Chakra:* heart

bond in relationships, disconnect: Amblygonite, Brandenberg Amethyst, Flint, Rainbow Mayanite, Shiva Lingam, Stibnite, Tugtupite, Wind Fossil Agate

bondage: Ajoite. *Chakra:* solar plexus

burn-out: Cobalto Calcite, Golden Healer Quartz, Lilac Quartz. *Chakra:* heart

catharsis, induce: Barite, Serpentine in Obsidian, Tugtupite

Unless otherwise directed, apply crystal over organ or site of symptom, place on appropriate chakra, wear as jewellery, bathe with or take as a crystal essence.

conditioning: Clevelandite, Golden Healer Quartz, Drusy Golden Healer. *Chakra:* solar plexus, third eye

dependency: Cobalto Calcite. *Chakra:* base

debris: Ajoite, Pink Lemurian Seed, Rainbow Mayanite. *Chakra:* solar plexus

dysfunction: Chinese Red Phantom Quartz, Fenster Quartz, Orange Kyanite. *Chakra:* higher heart

equilibrium: Adamite, Rutile with Hematite, Merlinite, Quantum Quattro, Shungite

exhaustion: Cinnabar in Jasper, Lilac Quartz, Orange River Quartz, Prehnite with Epidote

express: Blue Aragonite

frozen feelings: Clevelandite, Diopside, Eilat Stone, Ice Quartz, Scolecite. *Chakra:* solar plexus, heart, heart seed, higher heart

healing: Garnet in Quartz, Mount Shasta Opal, Tugtupite, Xenotine

hooks, remove: Amblygonite, Drusy Golden Healer, Golden Danburite, Goethite, Klinoptilolith, Novaculite, Nunderite, Nuummite, Orange Kyanite, Pyromorphite, Rainbow Mayanite, Tantalite, Tugtupite. *Chakra:* solar plexus

manipulation: Pink Lemurian Seed, Tantalite. *Chakra:* sacral, solar plexus, third eye

maturation: Alexandrite, Cobalto Calcite

negative, destructive attachments: Ajoite, Drusy Golden Healer, Ilmenite, Pink Lemurian Seed,

---

Unless otherwise directed, apply crystal over organ or site of symptom, place on appropriate chakra, wear as jewellery, bathe with or take as a crystal essence.

Rainbow Mayanite, Tantalite, Tinguaite. *Chakra:* base, solar plexus

pain after separation: Aegirine, Eilat Stone, Tugtupite. *Chakra:* higher heart

patterns: Arfvedsonite, Brandenberg Amethyst, Celadonite, Fenster Quartz, Rainbow Covellite, Scheelite. *Chakra:* solar plexus, base

recovery: Empowerite, Eye of the Storm, Lilac Quartz. *Chakra:* higher heart

release: Cobalto Calcite. *Chakra:* solar plexus, base, sacral

restore trust: Clevelandite, Faden Quartz, Xenotine

revitalize: Orange River Quartz, Vivianite

shock: Tugtupite, Tantalite. *Chakra:* heart

shut down, release: Ice Quartz

stability: Mohawkite. *Chakra:* base

stamina: Picrolite

strength: Brazilianite, Mohawkite, Picrolite, Tree Agate. *Chakra:* heart

stress: Cobalto Calcite, Eye of the Storm, Icicle Calcite, Shungite, Tugtupite. *Chakra:* solar plexus

tension: Strawberry Quartz. *Chakra:* solar plexus

toxicity: Ajoite, Arsenopyrite, Banded Agate, Champagne Aura Quartz, Drusy Danburite with Chlorite, Valentinite and Stibnite

trauma: Ajoite, Blue Euclase, Cobalto Calcite, Empowerite, Epidote, Gaia Stone, Graphic Smoky

Quartz (Zebra Stone), Holly Agate, Mangano Vesuvianite, Orange River Quartz, Richterite, Tantalite, Tugtupite, Victorite. *Chakra:* solar plexus
turmoil: Cobalto Calcite, Desert Rose. *Chakra:* base
underlying causes of distress: Eye of the Storm, Gaia Stone, Lemurian Gold Opal, Richterite, Riebekite with Sugilite and Bustamite, Smoky Amethyst. *Chakra:* solar plexus, past life
wounds: Ajoite, Bustamite, Cassiterite, Cobalto Calcite, Eilat Stone, Gaia Stone, Macedonian Opal, Mookaite Jasper, Orange River Quartz, Piemontite, Rathbunite™, Xenotine. *Chakra:* higher heart

Emphysema: Chrysotile, Chrysotile in Serpentine, Riebekite with Sugilite and Bustamite. *Chakra:* dantien

Empty nest syndrome: Menalite. *Chakra:* sacral

Endocrine system: Adamite, Amechlorite, Azeztulite with Morganite, Blue Quartz, Bustamite, Champagne Aura Quartz, Fire and Ice Quartz, Picrolite, Pink Heulandite, Richterite, Seriphos Quartz, Smoky Amethyst. *Chakra:* dantien, higher heart

Endometriosis: Blue Euclase, Vanadinite. *Chakra:* sacral

Endorphin release: Cavansite, Sillimanite. *Chakra:* alta major

Endurance, boost: Poppy Jasper. *Chakra:* base, sacral, dantien

Energy:
  amplify: Poppy Jasper, Preseli Bluestone, Ruby

Lavender Quartz. *Chakra:* base, dantien

depletion: Eudialyte, Macedonian Opal, Ruby Lavender Quartz, Pink Sunstone, Poppy Jasper, Preseli Bluestone, Que Sera, Ruby Lavender Quartz, Scheelite, Strawberry Lemurian. *Chakra:* dantien

energetic cleanse: Anandalite, Merlinite

field, strengthen: Mohawkite, Poppy Jasper, Preseli Bluestone, Ruby Lavender Quartz. *Chakra:* dantien, solar plexus

imbalances: Lepidocrosite

implants: Amechlorite, Cryolite, Drusy Golden Healer, Holly Agate, Ilmenite, Lemurian Aquitane Calcite, Novaculite, Nuummite, Rainbow Mayanite, Tantalite. *Chakra:* solar plexus, sacral

leakage from aura: Flint, Molybdenite in Quartz, Nuummite, Pyrite in Quartz, Strawberry Lemurian, Rainbow Mayanite, Tantalite. *Chakra:* dantien, higher heart

patterns: Celadonite, Schalenblende

system: Garnet in Quartz. *Chakra:* dantien

transfer: Phlogopite

unbalanced field: Garnet in Quartz, Preseli Bluestone

vampirisation: Gaspeite, Iridescent Pyrite, Nunderite, Tantalite, Xenotine and see Spleen chakra page 81

Endurance: Honey Phantom Calcite, Septarian. *Chakra:* base, sacral, dantien

Entities, remove attached: Drusy Golden Healer,

Klinoptilolith, Larvikite, Nirvana Quartz, Phantom Selenite, Pyromorphite, Rainbow Mayanite, Smoky Amethyst, Stibnite. *Chakra:* sacral, solar plexus, third eye

Environmental:

> **diseases:** Drusy Quartz on Sphalerite, Petrified Wood, Smoky Elestial Quartz, Shungite. *Chakra:* earth star (or place in environment)
>
> **pollution:** Alunite, Champagne Aura Quartz, Poppy Jasper, Smoky Elestial Quartz, Phlogopite, Que Sera, Shungite, Tantalite, Thunder Egg, Trummer Jasper. *Chakra:* earth star (place stones in earth or around house)
>
> **harmony:** Khutnohorite

Envy, ameliorate: Blood of Isis. *Chakra:* solar plexus, heart

Enzymes: Bixbite, Phlogopite, Shungite

Epilepsy: Astrophyllite, Dogtooth Calcite, Goethite, Pyrite in Magnesite, Scolecite. *Chakra:* dantien, third eye

Eruptions on skin: Snakeskin Agate, Faden Quartz, Honey Calcite, Klinoptilolith, Riebekite with Sugilite and Bustamite, Sulphur in Quartz, Wind Fossil Agate

Etheric:

> **blueprint:** Andescine Labradorite, Angelinite, Astraline, Brandenberg Amethyst, Chrysotile, Elestial Quartz, Ethiopian Opal, Eye of the Storm, Flint, Girasol, Keyiapo, Khutnohorite, Lemurian Aquitane Calcite, Rhodozite, Ruby Lavender Quartz, Sanda

Rosa Azeztulite, Scheelite, Stellar Beam Calcite, Tangerine Dream Lemurian, Tantalite. *Chakra:* past life

body: Ethiopian Opal, Golden Selenite and see Aura page 58

pests: Cryolite, Tantalite and see Aura page 58

support: Eye of the Storm, Mohawkite, Tantalite, Tremolite, Winchite

surgery: Eisenkiesel, Libyan Gold Tektite, Rainbow Mayanite, Seriphos Quartz, Stibnite, Vera Cruz Amethyst

Ethnic conflict: Afghanite, Azeztulite with Morganite, Catlinite, Champagne Aura Quartz, Chinese Red Quartz, Fluorapatite, Trigonic Quartz, Tugtupite

Eustachian tubes, blocked: Celestite, Lapis Lazuli

Everyday reality, difficulty in dealing with: Blue Halite, Bornite, Cathedral Quartz, Dumortierite, Lepidocrosite, Marcasite, Neptunite, Pearl Spa Dolomite, Purpurite. *Chakra:* earth star, dantien (or wear continuously)

Examinations: Eclipse Stone

Excretion: Leopardskin Jasper, Malacholla, Specularite

Exhaustion: Cinnabar in Jasper, Judy's Jasper, Poppy Jasper, Prehnite with Epidote, Schalenblende. *Chakra:* sacral, base, dantien

Extraneous thoughts: Paraiba Tourmaline

Extremities, burning: Fluorapatite

Eyes: Blue Chalcedony, Biotite, Cat's Eye Quartz, Cavansite, Covellite, Fenster Quartz, Fluorapatite, Gaia

Unless otherwise directed, apply crystal over organ or site of symptom, place on appropriate chakra, wear as jewellery, bathe with or take as a crystal essence.

Stone, Galaxyite, Granite, Indicolite Quartz, Lazulite, Nuummite, Paraiba Tourmaline, Pink Granite, Rosophia, Schalenblende, Vivianite

astigmatism: Fenster Quartz (place over eyes or bathe eyes in alcohol-free crystal essence)

bloodshot: Blue Chalcedony (bathe in alcohol-free crystal essence)

cooling: Gaia Stone, Halite, Jamesonite, Paraiba Tourmaline

disease: Fenster Quartz, Pink Granite, Unakite, Vivianite

impurities, irritants in: Blue Chalcedony, Blue Halite, Fenster Quartz, Gaia Stone, Pink Granite, Vivianite

infection: Ruby Lavender Quartz, Richterite, Vivianite

iris: Lepidocrosite

macular degeneration: Quartz with Lepidolite

optic nerve: Eudialyte, Kakortokite. *Chakra:* third eye

retina: Schalenblende

soothe: Blue Chalcedony, Paraiba Tourmaline

strengthen muscles: Aegirine, Bustamite, Cat's Eye Quartz, Nzuri Moyo, Phlogopite

tired: Scapolite

weak: Fenster Quartz, Huebnerite, Mystic Topaz

Eyesight: Cat's Eye Quartz, Fenster Quartz, Holey Stone. *Chakra:* third eye

---

Unless otherwise directed, apply crystal over organ or site of symptom, place on appropriate chakra, wear as jewellery, bathe with or take as a crystal essence.

- F -

Facial pain: Blue Euclase, Bronzite, Cathedral Quartz, Eilat Stone, Flint, Rhodozite

Fallopian tubes: see Reproductive organs page 177

Family:

> **stress:** Candle Quartz, Chinese Red Quartz, Datolite, Eye of the Storm, Faden Quartz, Fairy Quartz, Glendonite, Mohave Turquoise, Riebekite with Sugilite and Bustamite, Shaman Quartz, Shungite, Spirit Quartz. *Chakra:* solar plexus
>
> **sense of belonging:** Polychrome Jasper. *Chakra:* earth star and base
>
> **ties:** Cat's Eye Quartz, Glendonite, Polychrome Jasper. *Chakra:* solar plexus

Fatigue: Apricot Quartz, Girasol, Poppy Jasper, Strawberry Lemurian, Quantum Quattro, Pyrite in Quartz. *Chakra:* base, sacral, dantien

Fatty acids: Bixbite

Fear: Blue Quartz, Cacoxenite, Carolite, Dumortierite, Hackmanite, Icicle Calcite, Leopardskin Jasper, Oceanite, Paraiba Tourmaline, Spectrolite, Tangerose, Tugtupite. *Chakra:* heart, solar plexus

> **abandonment or rejection:** Clevelandite, Rhodozaz
>
> **death:** Arsenopyrite
>
> **dirt and bacteria:** Frondellite
>
> **of failure:** Avalonite, Elestial Quartz

Unless otherwise directed, apply crystal over organ or site of symptom, place on appropriate chakra, wear as jewellery, bathe with or take as a crystal essence.

future: Rosophia

irrational: Revelation Stone

responsibility: Brazilianite, Hemimorphite, Ocean Jasper, Paraiba Tourmaline, Quantum Quattro

terrorist activity: Super 7

the unknown: Bastnasite

Feet: Bustamite, Petrified Wood, Quantum Quattro, Stromatolite, Zebra Stone

Female rites of passage: Blue Euclase, Menalite

Feng shui: Ammolite

Fertility, increase: Calcite Fairy Stone, Dragon Stone, Menalite, Orange Kyanite, Tree Agate, Tugtupite. *Chakra:* sacral, dantien

Fever, lower: Bismuth, Chalcopyrite, Eilat Stone, Gabbro, Honey Opal, Limonite, Macedonian Opal, Pounamou Jade, Pyrite in Magnesite, Sulphur in Quartz, Thompsonite (place stone over site of greatest heat, in front of left ear, on third eye or take as crystal essence)

Fibroids: Menalite. *Chakra:* sacral

Fibromyalgia: Tanzine Aura Quartz

Fibrous growths: Gabbro, Menalite. *Chakra:* sacral

Filtration system: Shungite. *Chakra:* dantien

Finger nails, strengthen: Bustamite, Pearl Spa Dolomite

'First aid': Eye of the Storm, Garnet in Quartz, Quantum Quattro, Que Sera, Richterite, Tantalite. *Chakra:* dantien, higher heart

Flexibility: Cavansite, Kimberlite

Flu: Honey Opal, Macedonian Opal, Que Sera, Quantum Quattro, Rainforest Jasper, Shungite. *Chakra:* higher heart

Fluids: Nunderite, Oligoclase. *Chakra:* dantien, solar plexus

> **excess:** Brochantite, Scheelite, Smoky Amethyst
>
> **imbalances:** Azeztulite with Morganite, Bastnasite, Eye of the Storm, Hackmanite, Mookaite Jasper, Nunderite, Oligoclase, Rainforest Jasper, Scheelite
>
> **retention:** Andean Opal, Bustamite, Chalcanthite, Diaspore (Zultanite), Hackmanite, Halite, Hanksite, Mookaite Jasper, Nunderite, Scheelite, Smoky Amethyst, Sonora Sunrise

Fluorite, dissipate excess: Champagne Aura Quartz, Cryolite

Food poisoning: Shungite

Forgetfulness: see Mind page 147. *Chakra:* third eye

Forgiveness: Diopside, Khutnohorite, Tugtupite. *Chakra:* higher heart

'Fountain of Youth': Andara Glass

Fractures: Creedite, Faden Quartz and see Bones page 68

Frailty: Erythrite. *Chakra:* dantien, higher heart

Freckles: Marcasite

Free radical damage: Brochantite, Diaspore (Zultanite), Klinoptilolith, Shungite. *Chakra:* higher heart

Fright: see Trauma page 198

Frigidity: Poppy Jasper. *Chakra:* sacral, base

Frozen shoulder: Ice Quartz, Scapolite

Unless otherwise directed, apply crystal over organ or site of symptom, place on appropriate chakra, wear as jewellery, bathe with or take as a crystal essence.

Frustration, overcome: Chinese Red Quartz, Poppy Jasper, Pyrite in Magnesite. *Chakra:* base, dantien

Fungal infection: Arsenopyrite, Budd Stone (African Jade), Covellite, Klinoptilolith, Proustite, Rainbow Covellite, Shungite, Tree Agate (bathe with crystal essence or place stone over site)

    oral: Thompsonite

Unless otherwise directed, apply crystal over organ or site of symptom, place on appropriate chakra, wear as jewellery, bathe with or take as a crystal essence.

- G -

Gall, excess: Huebnerite

Gall bladder: Aegirine, Bytownite, Empowerite, Epidote, Gaspeite, Golden Danburite, Kambaba Jasper, Pyrite in Magnesite, Shungite. *Chakra:* sacral, dantien

Gallstones: Gaspeite, Leopardskin Jasper, Pyrite in Magnesite, Shungite

Gastric disturbance causing insomnia: Hackmanite, Khutnohorite, Pyrite in Quartz, Shungite. *Chakra:* solar plexus

Gastric:

ulcer: Shungite. *Chakra:* solar plexus

upset: Shungite. *Chakra:* solar plexus

Gastritis: Shungite

Genetic:

disorders: Amblygonite, Brandenberg Amethyst, Montebrasite, Petrified Wood and see DNA page 97. *Chakra:* dantien, solar plexus, alta major

memory: Petrified Wood, Revelation Stone

Genitals: Menalite, Shiva Lingam, Violane. *Chakra:* base

Genital herpes: Conichalcite, Hemimorphite, Ouro Verde

Genocide: Catlinite

Geopathic stress: Eye of the Storm, Pyrite and Sphalerite, Riebekite with Sugilite and Bustamite, Shungite, Smoky Elestial, Smoky Amethyst, Thunder Egg and see

---

Unless otherwise directed, apply crystal over organ or site of symptom, place on appropriate chakra, wear as jewellery, bathe with or take as a crystal essence.

Electromagnetic pollution page 101. *Chakra:* earth star (place around corners of house)

Gingivitis: see Gums page 116

Glands: Mookaite Jasper, Paraiba Tourmaline. *Chakra:* dantien, throat

Glandular:

    disturbances: Bastnasite, Mookaite Jasper

    fever: Honey Opal, Paraiba Tourmaline. *Chakra:* throat

    swellings: Agrellite, Anandalite™, Blue Euclase

Glaucoma: Marialite, Scapolite, Tanzine Aura Quartz. *Chakra:* throat

Goddess: Gaia Stone, Menalite

Gout: Galaxyite, Rosophia

Grief: Aegirine, Ajo Quartz, Blue Drusy Quartz, Cobalto Calcite, Datolite, Diopside, Empowerite, Epidote, Girasol, Indicolite Quartz, Khutnohorite, Mangano Vesuvianite, Quantum Quattro. *Chakra:* higher heart

Ground spirit into matter: Aztee, Champagne Aura Quartz, Empowerite, Keyiapo, Khutnohorite, Mohawkite, Peanut Wood, Schalenblende, Serpentine in Obsidian, Steatite. *Chakra:* dantien, soma

Grounding: Ajo Quartz, Amphibole, Aztee, Blue Aragonite, Bronzite, Bustamite, Calcite Fairy Stone, Champagne Aura Quartz, Cloudy Quartz, Dalmatian Stone, Empowerite, Flint, Gabbro, Healer's Gold, Hematoid Calcite, Honey Phantom Quartz, Kambaba

Jasper, Lazulite, Lemurian Jade, Leopardskin Serpentine, Keyiapo, Libyan Gold Tektite, Limonite, Lemurian Seed, Marcasite, Merlinite, Mohawkite, Novaculite, Nunderite, Peanut Wood, Pearl Spa Dolomite, Petrified Wood, Poppy Jasper, Preseli Bluestone, Purpurite, Pyrite in Magnesite, Quantum Quattro, Rutile with Hematite, Schalenblende, Smoky Elestial Quartz, Smoky Herkimer, Steatite, Stromatolite, Serpentine in Obsidian. *Chakra:* base, earth star, dantien

Growths: Biotite, Champagne Aura Quartz, Gabbro, Klinoptilolith, Rosophia, and see Tumours page 198

Guilt: Astrophyllite, Catlinite, Eudialyte, Hackmanite, Hematoid Calcite, Leopardskin Jasper, Messina Quartz, Pumice, Quantum Quattro, Tugtupite. *Chakra:* solar plexus, higher heart

Gums: Stichtite, Titanite (Sphene)

Guru disconnection: Banded Agate, Rainbow Mayanite

- H -

Habits, overcome: Heulandite, Oligoclase, Purpurite. *Chakra:* solar plexus

Haemoglobin: Specularite

Haemorrhage: Quantum Quattro (place over site)

Hair: Granite, Riebekite with Sugilite and Bustamite. *Chakra:* crown (rinse with crystal essence or wear stones as earrings)

    alopecia: Epidote, Girasol, Phosphosiderite. *Chakra:* solar plexus – brings up underlying cause

    baldness: Chalcopyrite, Phosphosiderite

    growth, stimulate: Chalcopyrite (massage with stone, or rinse with crystal essence)

    loss: Girasol, Phosphosiderite

Hallucinations: Ocean Jasper, Picture Jasper. *Chakra:* third eye, crown

Hands: Stromatolite (hold or wear crystal)

    cold: Aragonite and see Raynaud's disease page 175

    swollen: Trigonic Quartz

Harmony, promote: Khutnohorite. *Chakra:* solar plexus, heart

Hay fever: Paraiba Tourmaline, Shungite

Head: Bowenite (New Jade), Granite

Headache: Amblygonite, Bustamite, Cathedral Quartz, Champagne Aura Quartz, Dumortierite, Greenlandite, Quantum Quattro, Pyrite in Magnesite, Rhodozite,

---

Unless otherwise directed, apply crystal over organ or site of symptom, place on appropriate chakra, wear as jewellery, bathe with or take as a crystal essence.

Sugilite. *Chakra:* third eye

blocked alta major chakra: Garnet in Pyroxene, Herderite, Orange Kyanite, Riebekite with Sugilite and Bustamite, and see Alta Major chakra page 77

emotional cause: Glendonite, Khutnohorite, Mangano Vesuvianite, Mount Shasta Opal, Tangerose

neck tension: Alexandrite, Blue Euclase, Blue Siberian Quartz, Blue Moonstone

negative environmental factors/electromagnetic stress: see Electromagnetic stress page 101

poor posture: Blue Moonstone (on base of skull)

third eye blocked: Afghanite, Ajo Blue Calcite, Candle Quartz, Chalcedony with Apophyllite, Herderite, Holly Agate, Khutnohorite, Riebekite with Sugilite and Bustamite, and see Third eye chakra page 82

upset stomach: Dumortierite, Khutnohorite

Healing crisis: Eye of the Storm, Quantum Quattro, Smoky Elestial Quartz. *Chakra:* dantien, higher heart

Healing the healer: Blue Lemurian, Eye of the Storm, Faden Quartz, Healer's Gold, Indicolite Quartz, Molybdenite, Ocean Jasper, Quantum Quattro, Septarian. *Chakra:* dantien, higher heart

Hearing: Ammolite, Budd Stone (African Jade), Kambaba Jasper, Leopardskin Serpentine, Peanut Wood, Stromatolite

disorders: Ammolite, Budd Stone (African Jade),

Smoky Amethyst, Snakeskin Agate

loss: Kambaba Jasper, Leopardskin Serpentine, Peanut Wood, Stromatolite

Heart: Adamite, Andean Blue Opal, Brandenberg Amethyst, Bustamite, Candle Quartz, Cocoxenite, Fiskenaesset Ruby, Garnet in Quartz, Golden Danburite, Green Diopside, Green Heulandite, Holly Agate, Khutnohorite, Merlinite, Picrolite, Prasiolite, Quantum Quattro, Rose Quartz Elestial, Rosophia, Tugtupite and see Heart chakra page 79. *Chakra:* heart

attack: Gaspeite, Tantalite, Tugtupite

beat, irregular: Dumortierite. *Chakra:* dantien

burn: Montebrasite, Pyrophyllite

broken: Candle Quartz, Cobalto Calcite, Creedite, Garnet in Granite, Khutnohorite, Roselite, Ruby in Granite, Ruby in Moonstone, Smoky Rose Quartz, Tugtupite

chakra: see Chakras page 79

disease: Hemimorphite, Smoky Amethyst

failure: Scheelite

healer: Azeztulite with Morganite, Khutnohorite, Pyroxmangite, Rhodozaz, Roselite, Rosophia

inflammation: Blue Euclase, Pink Lemurian Seed, Rhodozite, Sulphur in Quartz,

invigorate: Chohua Jasper, Lemurian Jade

muscle: Septarian

rhythm, disturbed: Brandenberg Amethyst

Unless otherwise directed, apply crystal over organ or site of symptom, place on appropriate chakra, wear as jewellery, bathe with or take as a crystal essence.

stabilize rhythm: Honey Calcite

strengthen: Chohua Jasper, Erythrite, Honey Calcite, Lemurian Jade, Pink Lemurian Seed, Strawberry Quartz

trauma: Azeztulite with Morganite, Blue Euclase, Cobalto Calcite, Gaia Stone, Mangano Vesuvianite, Oceanite, Peanut Wood, Quantum Quattro, Rose Quartz Elestial, Roselite, Ruby Lavender Quartz, Tantalite, Victorite

unblock: Gaspeite, Pink Lemurian Seed, Prasiolite, Smoky Rose Quartz

Heartache: Cobalto Calcite, Faden Quartz, Gaspeite, Honey Opal, Pink Crackle Quartz, Pink Lemurian Seed, Morion, Roselite. *Chakra:* higher heart

Heart seed chakra: see Chakras page 76

Heatstroke: Rose or Smoky Elestial Quartz

Heavy metals, mobilize: Apple Aura Quartz, Brazilianite, Chinese Chromium Quartz, Klinoptilolith, Orange River Quartz, Shungite. *Chakra:* spleen

Helplessness: Actinolite Quartz, Adamite, Brazilianite, Bronzite, Clevelandite, Covellite, Dumortierite, Ocean Jasper, Kakortokite, Mystic Topaz, Paraiba Tourmaline, Pumice, Quantum Quattro, Tree Agate. *Chakra:* earth star, base, sacral, dantien

Hernia: Bastnasite, Mookaite Jasper, Stichtite

Herpes: Conichalcite, Ouro Verde. *Chakra:* throat

Hiatus hernia: Goethite (tape over site)

Unless otherwise directed, apply crystal over organ or site of symptom, place on appropriate chakra, wear as jewellery, bathe with or take as a crystal essence.

Higher heart chakra: see Chakras page 76

Higher mind, align: Amethyst Herkimer, Auralite 23, Goethite, Hackmanite, Herderite, Sacred Scribe (Russian Lemurian), Septarian, Sillimanite, Yellow Phantom Quartz. *Chakra:* third eye

Higher self, contact: Amphibole, Anandalite, Anthrophyllite, Bushman Red Cascade Quartz, Cathedral Quartz, Faden Quartz, Fire and Ice Quartz, Golden Healer Quartz, Green Ridge Quartz, Mangano Vesuvianite, Porphyrite (Chinese Letter Stone), Prasiolite, Orange River Quartz, Rosophia, Sugar Blade Quartz, Ussingite

High blood pressure: see Blood pressure page 66

High vibrational downloads, ground and harmonize: Agnitite™, Ajo Quartz, Anandalite™, Angelsite, Aurichalcite, Aztee, Bismuth, Empowerite, Golden Healer Quartz, Lemurian Gold Opal, Petrified Wood, Phosphosiderite, Rosophia, Ruby Lavender Quartz, Sanda Rosa Azeztulite, Victorite. *Chakra:* dantien, soma

Hippocampus: Blue Moonstone, Preseli Bluestone. *Chakra:* alta major

Hips, pain: Blue Euclase, Bronzite, Cathedral Quartz, Eilat Stone, Flint, Khutnohorite, Quantum Quattro, Rhodozite, Serpentine in Obsidian, Smoky Amethyst, Spider Web Obsidian

HIV/AIDs: Catlinite, Diaspore, Petoskey Stone, Schalenblende, Scheelite, Sonora Sunrise, Shungite.

Unless otherwise directed, apply crystal over organ or site of symptom, place on appropriate chakra, wear as jewellery, bathe with or take as a crystal essence.

Chakra: dantien, higher heart

Hoarseness: Crystalline Kyanite, Hackmanite. *Chakra:* throat

Homeostasis: Enstatite and Diopside, Klinoptilolith, Piemontite, Reinerite. *Chakra:* dantien

Homophobia: Oceanite, Zircon

Honesty, with self: Bumble Bee Jasper, Rosophia

'Hooks', removing: Drusy Golden Healer, Goethite, Klinoptilolith, Nunderite, Orange Kyanite, Pyromorphite, Rainbow Mayanite, Tantalite. *Chakra:* sacral, solar plexus, third eye

Hormones:

    boosting: Amechlorite, Cassiterite, Menalite, Paraiba Tourmaline, Smoky Amethyst. *Chakra:* third eye, higher heart

    imbalances: Amechlorite, Astrophyllite, Black Moonstone, Champagne Aura Quartz, Chinese Chromium Quartz, Diopside, Hemimorphite, Menalite, Paraiba Tourmaline, Sonora Sunrise, Tanzine Aura Quartz, Tugtupite. *Chakra:* third eye, higher heart

    regulate: Champagne Aura Quartz, Chinese Chromium Quartz, Menalite, Smoky Amethyst, Tugtupite. *Chakra:* third eye, higher heart

Hospitalization: Poppy Jasper

Hot flashes/flushes: Crackled Fire Agate, Gabbro, Menalite

Unless otherwise directed, apply crystal over organ or site of symptom, place on appropriate chakra, wear as jewellery, bathe with or take as a crystal essence.

Hyperactivity: Cumberlandite, Dianite, Fiskenaesset Ruby, Lepidocrosite, Montebrasite, Pearl Spa Dolomite, Yellow Scapolite. *Chakra:* earth star, base, dantien

Hypersensitivity: Dumortierite, Proustite and see Oversensitive page 158

Hyperthyroidism: Cacoxenite, Champagne Aura Quartz, Cryolite, Richterite, Tanzine Aura Quartz. *Chakra:* throat Quartz (or wear continuously)

Hypoglycaemia: Atlantasite, Bowenite (New Jade), Datolite, Maw Sit Sit, Pink Opal, Schalenblende, Stichtite and Serpentine, Tugtupite and see Pancreas page 159. *Chakra:* dantien, spleen

Hypothalamus: Blue Moonstone, Preseli Bluestone, Richterite, Tanzine Aura Quartz

Hysterectomy: Menalite

Hysteria: Marcasite. *Chakra:* solar plexus

'Identified patient'/takes on the family pain or dis-ease:
Fenster Quartz, Polychrome Jasper

Idleness, overcome: Poppy Jasper. *Chakra:* base, dantien

Ill-wishing: Crackled Fire Agate, Limonite, Master Shamanite, Mohawkite, Nunderite, Nuummite, Purpurite, Richterite, Tantalite, Tugtupite. *Chakra:* throat (wear continuously)

Illusions:

assess: Larvikite, Rosophia

dispel: Adularia, Fairy Wand Quartz, Lemurian Seed, Lepidocrosite, Ilmenite, Kornerupine, Neptunite, Nirvana Quartz, Quartz with Mica, Vivianite

Immune system: Amechlorite, Anandalite™, Diaspore (Zultanite), Klinoptilolith, Lemurian Jade, Macedonian Opal, Mookaite Jasper, Nzuri Moyo, Ocean Jasper, Paraiba Tourmaline, Petrified Wood, Preseli Bluestone, Quantum Quattro, Que Sera, Richterite, Rosophia, Seriphos Quartz, Shungite, Smoky Quartz with Aegerine, Super 7, Winchite. *Chakra:* dantien, higher heart

Impacted vertebrae: Calcite Fairy Quartz, Huebnerite and see Spine page 187

Implants: Ajoite, Amechlorite, Cryolite, Drusy Golden Healer, Holly Agate, Ilmenite, Lemurian Aquitane Calcite, Novaculite, Nuummite, Rainbow Mayanite, Tantalite. *Chakra:* crown

---

Unless otherwise directed, apply crystal over organ or site of symptom, place on appropriate chakra, wear as jewellery, bathe with or take as a crystal essence.

Imposter syndrome: Rhodozaz. *Chakra:* dantien

Impotence: Bastnasite, Rutile, Shiva Lingam, Shungite. *Chakra:* base, sacral

Inadequacy: Eye of the Storm, Poppy Jasper, Pumice. *Chakra:* dantien

Incarnation, ameliorate discomfort in: Ajo Blue Calcite, Celestobarite, Empowerite, Guardian Stone, Keyiapo, Orange Kyanite, Peanut Wood, Pearl Spar Dolomite, Polychrome Jasper, Red Celestial Quartz, Riebekite with Sugilite and Bustamite, Rosophia, Sanda Rosa Azeztulite, Snakeskin Agate, Strontianite, Thompsonite. *Chakra:* soma, dantien and earth star

Incest, overcome effects: Cobalto Calcite, Eilat Stone, Tugtupite. *Chakra:* base, sacral, solar plexus (wear continuously, or place over chakras for 20 minutes daily)

Incontinence: Peanut Wood, Petrified Wood, Scapolite. *Chakra:* sacral, dantien

Indigestion: Cryolite, Pyrophyllite, Steatite. *Chakra:* solar plexus

Indigo/crystal/rainbow/star children: Cat's Eye Quartz, Sanda Rosa Azeztulite, Stichtite, Tremolite, Youngite

Indulgence, overcome effects of: Brandenberg Amethyst, Vera Cruz Amethyst (wear continuously)

Infection: Gabbro, Quantum Quattro, Que Sera, Richterite, Ruby Lavender Quartz, Shungite, Tree Agate. *Chakra:* higher heart

    increase resistance to: Quantum Quattro, Que Sera,

Unless otherwise directed, apply crystal over organ or site of symptom, place on appropriate chakra, wear as jewellery, bathe with or take as a crystal essence.

Shungite (wear continuously)

Infectious illness: Quantum Quattro, Que Sera, Shungite. *Chakra:* higher heart

Infertility: Banded Agate, Bastnasite, Bixbite, Blue Euclase, Brookite, Citrine Herkimer, Fiskenaesset Ruby, Granite, Menalite, Shiva Lingam, Spirit Quartz, Tugtupite. *Chakra:* sacral

   arising from infection: Menalite, Shungite

Inferiority complex: Pyrite in Magnesite. *Chakra:* dantien

Inflammation: Blue Euclase, Chalcopyrite, Dianite, Diopside, Hanksite, Ocean Jasper, Rhodozite, Sulphur in Quartz

   bladder and intestinal: Bastnasite, Gaspeite, Honey Calcite, Scheelite

   kidneys: Brazilianite, Diopside, Klinoptilolith, Nunderite, White Chohua Jasper

   joints: Dianite, Petrified Wood, Nzuri Moyo, Sulphur in Quartz, Tantalite

   skin: Chrysotile in Serpentine, Honey Calcite, Riebekite with Sugilite and Bustamite

   urethra: Scheelite

Influenza: Cathedral Quartz, Quantum Quattro, Que Sera, Shungite. *Chakra:* higher heart

Inhibitions: Poppy Jasper. *Chakra:* base

Inner child: Cobalto Calcite, Dalmatian Stone, Fairy Quartz, Hanksite, Limonite, Pink Crackle Quartz, Quantum Quattro, Spirit Quartz, Voegesite, Youngite.

Unless otherwise directed, apply crystal over organ or site of symptom, place on appropriate chakra, wear as jewellery, bathe with or take as a crystal essence.

Chakra: sacral

Inorgasmia: Orange Kyanite, Rutile, Shiva Lingam. *Chakra:* base, sacral, dantien

Insect bites: Klinoptilolith, Shungite

Insecurity: Leopardskin Jasper. *Chakra:* base

Institutionalised: Bismuth

Insomnia: Khutnohorite, Mount Shasta Opal, Pink Sunstone, Poldervaarite, Rosophia, Shungite (place by the bed or under the pillow)

> **disturbed sleep patterns:** Khutnohorite, Owyhee Blue Opal, Petrified Wood
>
> **emotional cause:** Glendonite, Khutnohorite, Mangano Vesuvianite, Mount Shasta Opal, Tangerose
>
> **geopathic/electromagnetic stress/pollution:** Eye of the Storm, Gabbro, Klinoptilolith, Shungite, Smoky Herkimer Diamond, Thunder Egg (place round bed or around the four corners of the room or house, depending on how strong the stress)
>
> **mental overload:** Crystal Cap Amethyst, Guinea Fowl Jasper, Red Amethyst, Spectrolite
>
> **negative environmental influences:** Champagne Aura Quartz, Elestial Smoky Quartz, Klinoptilolith, Shungite, Tantalite, Trummer Jasper (place around the four corners of the room)
>
> **nightmares/night terrors:** Spirit Quartz, Fairy Quartz, Dalmatian Stone, Tremolite. *Chakra:* third eye
>
> **overactive mind:** Auralite 23, Bytownite, Crystal Cap

Amethyst, Rhodozite, Spectrolite. *Chakra:* third eye

psychic overload: Auralite 23, Red Amethyst, Spectrolite. *Chakra:* third eye

stress: Eye of the Storm, Lemurian Gold Opal, Riebekite with Sugilite and Bustamite, Shungite and see Stress page 190. *Chakra:* higher heart

Insults, turn away: Bronzite, Tantalite. *Chakra:* higher heart

Insulin regulation: Astraline, Candle Quartz, Maw Sit Sit, Malacholla, Nuummite, Pink Opal, Red Serpentine, Schalenblende, Serpentine in Obsidian, Shungite and see Blood sugar page 67 and Pancreas page 159. *Chakra:* spleen, dantien

Integrity: Porphyrite (Chinese Letter Stone)

Intellect:

    improve: Blue Quartz, Porphyrite (Chinese Letter Stone). *Chakra:* third eye, crown

    stabilize: Ammolite, Septarian. *Chakra:* third eye, crown

Intercellular:

    blockages: Gold in Quartz, Golden Healer Quartz, Plancheite, Pyrite and Sphalerite, Rainbow Mayanite, Rhodozite, Serpentine in Obsidian

    structures: Ajo Blue Calcite, Candle Quartz, Cradle of Life, Gold in Quartz, Golden Healer Quartz, Lemurian Aquitane Calcite, Messina Quartz, Quantum Quattro, Que Sera, Pollucite, Rhodozite

Unless otherwise directed, apply crystal over organ or site of symptom, place on appropriate chakra, wear as jewellery, bathe with or take as a crystal essence.

Interface:

   communication with higher beings: Anandalite, Angels Wing Calcite, Lemurian Aquitane Calcite, Mohawkite, Trigonic Amethyst, Trigonic Quartz. *Chakra:* soma, soul star, stellar gateway

   healer and client: Andescine Labradorite, Brochantite, Healer's Gold, Iridescent Pyrite, Lemurian Jade, Master Shamanite, Mohawkite, Nunderite, Richterite, Scheelite, Serpentine in Obsidian, Spectrolite, Tantalite. *Chakra:* spleen

   self and outside world: Andescine Labradorite, Healer's Gold, Lemurian Jade, Mohawkite, Master Shamanite, Nunderite, Richterite, Serpentine in Obsidian, Spectrolite, Tantalite. *Chakra:* spleen, dantien

Internal organs: Ocean Jasper. *Chakra:* dantien

Intestines: Eclipse Stone, Empowerite, Honey Calcite, Merlinite. *Chakra:* dantien

   activate: Basalt

   small: Merlinite, Septarian. *Chakra:* sacral

   large: Astrophyllite

   lower: Rosophia

Intestinal disorders: Bastnasite, Bismuth, Cryolite, Gaspeite, Halite, Hanksite, Honey Calcite, Scolecite, Septarian. *Chakra:* sacral, dantien

Intimacy, lack of: Axinite, Datolite, Tugtupite

Intolerance: Pyrite in Magnesite

Unless otherwise directed, apply crystal over organ or site of symptom, place on appropriate chakra, wear as jewellery, bathe with or take as a crystal essence.

Introspection: Amphibole Quartz, Steatite. *Chakra:* third eye

Intuitive vision: Amphibole, Anandalite, Auralite 23, Blue Euclase, Bytownite, Tangerine Aura Quartz, Tanzanite, Tanzine Aura Quartz, Blue Selenite, and see Third eye chakra page 82. *Chakra:* third eye, crown

Involuntary movements, twitches: Fenster Quartz

Iris: see Eyes page 108

Iron:

> **excess:** Huebnerite
>
> **malabsorption:** Bronzite, Green Ridge Quartz, Limonite, Vivianite. *Chakra:* base

Irritable bowel syndrome (IBS): Amblygonite, Bastnasite, Cryolite, Montebrasite, Pumice, Rosophia, Scolecite, Xenotine. *Chakra:* dantien

Irritability: Fluorapatite, Pyrite in Magnesite. *Chakra:* base, sacral, dantien

Irritant filter: Pumice. *Chakra:* dantien

- J -

Jaw pain: Blue Euclase, Flint, Molybdenite, Paraiba Tourmaline, Quantum Quattro, Rhodozite

Jaundice: Holly Agate, Limonite

Jealousy: Eclipse Stone, Heulandite, Rainbow Mayanite, Rosophia, Tugtupite, Zircon. *Chakra:* heart

Jet lag: Preseli Bluestone, Proustite, Thunder Egg (wear or sip crystal essence frequently)

Joints: Cat's Eye Quartz, Messina Quartz, Petrified Wood, Phantom Calcite, Poldervaarite, Rhodozite

    calcified: Bornite, Calcite Fairy Stone, Prophecy Stone, Strontianite

    compressed: Graphic Smoky Quartz (Zebra Stone), Tantalite

    flexibility: Bastnasite, Cavansite, Kimberlite, Prehnite with Epidote, Peach Selenite, Selenite Phantom, Strontianite

    inflammation: Nzuri Moyo, Peach Selenite, Rhodozite, Sulphur in Quartz

    mobilize: Aztee, Calcite Fairy Stone, Nzuri Moyo, Petrified Wood, Prehnite with Epidote, Strontianite

    pain: Blue Euclase, Champagne Aura Quartz, Cathedral Quartz, Flint, Eilat Stone, Khutnohorite, Nzuri Moyo, Quantum Quattro, Rhodozite, Tantalite

    strengthening: Clevelandite, Tantalite

    swollen: Nzuri Moyo, Trigonic Quartz

Unless otherwise directed, apply crystal over organ or site of symptom, place on appropriate chakra, wear as jewellery, bathe with or take as a crystal essence.

Journeying: Aztee, Andean Opal, Polychrome Jasper, Preseli Bluestone, Scolecite, Sedona Stone, Serpentine in Obsidian, Titanite (Sphene) and see Shamanic journey page 182

Judgementalism: Green Heulandite, Mohawkite, Tantalite. *Chakra:* dantien

---

Unless otherwise directed, apply crystal over organ or site of symptom, place on appropriate chakra, wear as jewellery, bathe with or take as a crystal essence.

- K -

Karma:

burn off: Chinese Red Quartz and see Past life healing page 162

of grace, invoke: Wind Fossil Agate

Karmic:

blueprint: Cloudy Quartz, Keyiapo, Khutnohorite, Rhodozite, Ruby Lavender Quartz, Sanda Rosa Azeztulite, Scheelite, Titanite (Sphene)

cleansing: Cloudy Quartz, Holly Agate, Lemurian Seed, Wind Fossil Agate

contracts: Boli Stone, Gabbro, Leopardskin Jasper, Red Amethyst, Wind Fossil Agate

codependency: Quantum Quattro, Xenotine

debris: Nuummite, Peach Selenite, Rainbow Mayanite, Smoky Spirit Quartz, Wind Fossil Agate. *Chakra:* past life

debts: Holly Agate, Nuummite. *Chakra:* past life

dis-ease: Covellite, Isis Calcite, Nuummite and see Past life page 160. *Chakra:* past life

enmeshment: Smoky Elestial Quartz

emotional healing: Porphyrite (Chinese Letter Stone), Tangerose

entanglements: Flint, Novaculite, Nuummite, Peach Selenite, Rainbow Mayanite

family burdens: Mohawkite, Polychrome Jasper,

Unless otherwise directed, apply crystal over organ or site of symptom, place on appropriate chakra, wear as jewellery, bathe with or take as a crystal essence.

Tinguaite

healing: Andean Opal, Merlinite, Violane and see Past life healing page 162

wounds: Ajoite, Ajo Quartz, Green Ridge Quartz, Lemurian Seed, Macedonian Opal, Mookaite Jasper, Rathbunite™, Rosophia, Scheelite, Xenotine

Kidneys: Bastnasite, Black Moonstone, Brookite, Conichalcite, Blue Quartz, Chohua Jasper, Diopside, Fiskenaesset Ruby, Gaspeite, Heulandite, Leopardskin Jasper, Libyan Gold Tektite, Nunderite, Nuummite, Prehnite with Epidote, Quantum Quattro, Shungite, Serpentine in Obsidian, Sonora Sunrise, Stromatolite, Tanzanite. *Chakra:* dantien, solar plexus

cleanse: Brazilianite, Eye of the Storm (Judy's Jasper), Fire and Ice Quartz, Klinoptilolith, Nuummite, Prehnite with Epidote

degeneration: Quantum Quattro, Rosophia

detoxify: Amechlorite, Chohua Jasper, Eye of the Storm, Fire and Ice Quartz, Fiskenaesset Ruby, Kambaba Jasper, Klinoptilolith, Larvikite, Leopardskin Jasper, Nuummite, Quantum Quattro, Pyrite in Magnesite, Rainbow Covellite, Richterite, Shungite, Smoky Quartz with Aegerine

fortify: Heulandite

infections: Fiskenaesset Ruby, Libyan Gold Tektite, Richterite

regulating: Lemurian Jade

Unless otherwise directed, apply crystal over organ or site of symptom, place on appropriate chakra, wear as jewellery, bathe with or take as a crystal essence.

stimulating: Quantum Quattro, Septarian

stones: Calcite Fairy Stone, Flint, Pyrite in Magnesite

Kinesiology: Preseli Bluestone

Knees: Spider Web Obsidian

Kundalini: Agnitite™, Anandalite™, Bowenite (New Jade), Brazilianite, Chohua Jasper, Dragon Stone, Flame Aura Quartz, Garnet in Quartz, Kundalini Quartz, Serpentine in Obsidian, Stichtite, Victorite. *Chakra:* base

uncontrolled: Stichtite and Serpentine. *Chakra:* base, sacral

Unless otherwise directed, apply crystal over organ or site of symptom, place on appropriate chakra, wear as jewellery, bathe with or take as a crystal essence.

- L -

Lactation: Rutile, Stone of Dreams
   impaired: Menalite, Rutile
   improve: Menalite
Labour pains: Ammolite, Blue Euclase, Cathedral Quartz, Menalite, Quantum Quattro, Rhodozite. *Chakra:* sacral, dantien
Larynx: Crystalline Kyanite, Indicolite Quartz. *Chakra:* throat
Laryngitis: Shungite. *Chakra:* throat (wear continuously over site or gargle with crystal essence)
Learning difficulties: Annabergite. *Chakra:* third eye, crown, alta major
Left-right confusion: Bustamite with Sugilite. *Chakra:* third eye, crown, alta major
Legs: Bustamite
   restless: Hemimorphite
Leprosy: Snakeskin Agate
Lethargy: Apricot Quartz, Brookite, Golden Selenite, Orange Drusy Quartz, Pink Sunstone, Realgar and Orpiment, Sedona Stone, Tantalite. *Chakra:* base, sacral, dantien
Letting go past: Axinite, Fenster Quartz, Fulgarite, Green Diopside, Kimberlite, Lepidocrosite, Kakortokite, Nuummite, Paraiba Tourmaline, Pumice, Scheelite, Zircon. *Chakra:* solar plexus, heart, past life

---

Unless otherwise directed, apply crystal over organ or site of symptom, place on appropriate chakra, wear as jewellery, bathe with or take as a crystal essence.

Leukaemia: Alexandrite

Libido: Crackled Fire Agate, Eudialyte, Kundalini Quartz, Orange Kyanite, Poppy Jasper, Shungite, Sonora Sunrise, Tangerose, Tiffany Stone. *Chakra:* base, sacral

Life force, increase: Crackled Fire Agate, Libyan Gold Tektite, Moldau Quartz, Poppy Jasper. *Chakra:* higher heart, dantien (or wear continuously)

Life purpose: Cobalto Calcite, Victorite and see Soul plan page 184

Life support: Eye of the Storm. *Chakra:* dantien, higher heart

Ligaments, torn: Creedite

Lightbody: Agnitite™, Anandalite™, Golden Coracalcite, Golden Healer Quartz, Golden Himalayan Azeztulite, Mahogany Sheen Obsidian, Nirvana Quartz, Prophecy Stone, Rainbow Mayanite, Satyaloka Quartz, Satyamani Quartz, Scolecite, Sugar Blade Quartz, Trigonic Quartz, Vera Cruz Amethyst. *Chakra:* soma, higher crown

Lightworkers: Lemurian Seed, Rainbow Mayanite, Trigonic Quartz

Light-headedness: Celestobarite, Smoky Elestial Quartz, Victorite *Chakra:* dantien

Limiting patterns of behaviour: Ajoite, Amphibole, Atlantasite, Arfvedsonite, Barite, Botswana Agate, Bronzite, Cassiterite, Celadonite, Crackled Fire Agate, Chlorite Shaman Quartz, Dalmatian Stone, Datolite,

Unless otherwise directed, apply crystal over organ or site of symptom, place on appropriate chakra, wear as jewellery, bathe with or take as a crystal essence.

Dream Quartz, Dumortierite, Epidote, Garnet in Quartz, Glendonite, Hematoid Calcite, Halite, Hanksite, Honey Phantom Calcite, Indicolite Quartz, Kinoite, Marcasite, Merlinite, Nuummite, Oligoclase, Owyhee Blue Opal, Pearl Spa Dolomite, Porphyrite (Chinese Letter Stone), Quantum Quattro, Rainbow Covellite, Scheelite, Spider Web Obsidian, Stellar Beam Calcite. *Chakra:* base, sacral, dantien, solar plexus, past life

Linguistic capability: Annabergite, Calligraphy Stone, Chinese Writing Stone, Dumortierite, Novaculite. *Chakra:* throat, third eye, soma

Liver: Black Moonstone, Brookite, Cinnabar in Jasper, Empowerite, Gaspeite, Golden Danburite, Eilat Stone, Epidote, Guinea Fowl Jasper, Huebnerite, Heulandite, Lazulite, Lepidocrosite, Limonite, Poppy Jasper, Orange River Quartz, Red Amethyst, Shungite, Tugtupite. *Chakra:* dantien

> **blockages:** Bastnasite, Gaspeite, Holly Agate, Orange Kyanite, Poppy Jasper, Rhodozite
>
> **blood flow:** Mookaite Jasper
>
> **cleanse:** Crystal Cap Amethyst, Gaspeite, Klinoptilolith
>
> **depletion:** Holly Agate, Macedonian Opal, Tugtupite
>
> **detoxifying:** Amechlorite, Bastnasite, Eye of the Storm, Gaspeite, Kambaba Jasper, Klinoptilolith, Larvikite, Mtrolite, Pyrite in Magnesite, Rainbow Covellite, Richterite, Shungite, Smoky Quartz with

Aegerine

spots: Snakeskin Agate

stimulate: Poppy Jasper, Tugtupite

Longevity: Ammolite

Lower-back problems: see Back page 62

Lower limbs: Heulandite

Love: Cobalto Calcite, Elestial Rose Quartz, Khutnohorite, Rose Aura Quartz, Tugtupite. *Chakra:* heart, heart seed, higher heart

    accepting: Mystic Topaz, Tugtupite

    and spirituality: Smoky Rose Quartz

    attract: Alexandrite, Blue Aragonite, Strawberry Quartz, Twin Flame formation

    bond: Datolite, Erythrite, Eudialyte

    combine logic with: Seriphos Quartz

    compassionate: Bixbite, Candle Quartz, Mangano Vesuvianite, Tugtupite

    desperate for: Pink Halite, Quantum Quattro, Tugtupite

    enhance: Bornite on Silver

    fear around: Avalonite, Tangerose, Tugtupite

    for oneself: Dumortierite, Elestial Rose Quartz, Eudialyte, Faden Quartz, Gaia Stone, Lepidocrosite, Rose Aura Quartz, Tangerose, Titanite (Sphene), Tugtupite

    increase capacity to: Candle Quartz, Strawberry Quartz, Tugtupite

---

inner divine: Candle Quartz, Faden Quartz, Strawberry Quartz, Tugtupite. *Chakra:* third eye, crown

mature: Greenlandite

mutual: Datolite, Stellar Beam Calcite, Tugtupite

non-smothering: Botswana Agate

old, cut the cords of: Lemurian Aquitane Calcite, Novaculite, Nunderite, Nuummite, Rainbow Mayanite. *Chakra:* solar plexus, sacral, past life

open to possibility of: Mystic Topaz, Quantum Quattro, Tugtupite

parent-child: Tugtupite

promotion of: Candle Quartz

reawaken: Fiskenaesset Ruby

tough love: Cassiterite

transform psychic attack into: Tugtupite. *Chakra:* higher heart

unconditional: Cobalto Calcite, Crystalline Kyanite, Gaia Stone, Lemurian Seed, Poldervaarite, Rose Aura Quartz, Smoky Rose Quartz, Tangerine Aura, Tiffany Stone, Tugtupite, Zircon. *Chakra:* higher heart

universal: Ajoite, Amphibole, Anandalite, Brandenberg Amethyst, Drusy Quartz, Pink Lemurian Seed, Spirit Quartz, Vera Cruz Amethyst

Lucid dreaming: Dream Quartz, Scolecite

shield during: Azotic Topaz, Aztee, Bowenite (New Jade), Crackled Fire Agate, Gabbro, Lorenzenite

---

Unless otherwise directed, apply crystal over organ or site of symptom, place on appropriate chakra, wear as jewellery, bathe with or take as a crystal essence.

(Ramsayite), Master Shamanite, Mohave Turquoise, Mohawkite, Morion, Polychrome Jasper, Pyromorphite, Red Amethyst, Schalenblende, Silver Leaf Jasper, Tantalite, Thunder Egg

Lungs: Adamite, Ammolite, Andean Blue Opal, Blue Aragonite, Blue Quartz, Bustamite, Cacoxenite, Catlinite, Diopside, Fluorapatite, Graphic Smoky Quartz (Zebra Stone), Greenlandite, Kambaba Jasper, Petrified Wood, Prehnite with Epidote, Quantum Quattro, Scolecite, Serpentine in Obsidian, Smoky Amethyst, Sonora Sunrise, Tremolite, Valentinite and Stibnite. *Chakra:* dantien, higher heart

> **congested:** Vanadinite, Moss Agate
> **difficulty in breathing:** Anthrophyllite, Green Siberian Quartz, Riebekite with Sugilite and Bustamite, Tremolite and see Breathlessness page 71
> **fluid in:** Hackmanite, Halite, Hanksite, Ocean Jasper, Scheelite, Smoky Amethyst

Lupus: Chinese Red Quartz, Eudialyte

Lymphatic system: Anglesite, Bastnasite, Eye of the Storm (Judy's Jasper), Graphic Smoky Quartz, Hackmanite, Lazulite, Ocean Blue Jasper, Scheelite, Shungite, Trigonic Quartz, Zebra Stone. *Chakra:* dantien, higher heart

> **cleansing:** Bastnasite, Crystal Cap Amethyst, Feather Pyrite, Ocean Jasper
> **infections:** Shungite

Unless otherwise directed, apply crystal over organ or site of symptom, place on appropriate chakra, wear as jewellery, bathe with or take as a crystal essence.

stimulating: Ocean Jasper, Oligoclase

swellings: Agrellite, Anandalite™, Blue Euclase, Crystal Cap Amethyst

Unless otherwise directed, apply crystal over organ or site of symptom, place on appropriate chakra, wear as jewellery, bathe with or take as a crystal essence.

- M -

Macular degeneration: see Eyes page 108

Magnesium absorption: see Absorption page 50. *Chakra:* solar plexus

Malaria: Rainforest Jasper

Male-female imbalance: Shiva Lingam and see Yin-yang page 207. *Chakra:* sacral, dantien

Malignant conditions: Klinoptilolith, Quantum Quattro, Shungite

Malnutrition: Cassiterite

Mania: Novaculite. *Chakra:* dantien

Marfan syndrome: Kornerupine

Martyrdom: Cassiterite, Epidote, Prasiolite, Tugtupite. *Chakra:* higher heart, solar plexus

Maternal instinct: Menalite, Tugtupite. *Chakra:* base, sacral

ME: Chinese Red Quartz, Quantum Quattro, Que Sera, Shungite. *Chakra:* dantien

Measles: Dalmatian Stone

Meditative states, enter easily: Anandalite, Bytownite, Blue Selenite, Golden Azeztulite, Lemurian Seed, Pink Petalite. *Chakra:* third eye, crown

Membranes, inflamed: Hanksite

Memory:

> **improve:** Barite, Coprolite, Hematoid Calcite, Herderite, Klinoptilolith, Marcasite, Phantom Calcite,

Pyrite and Sphalerite, Vivianite. *Chakra:* third eye, crown

suppressed: Revelation Stone

Ménières disease: Ammolite, Quantum Quattro (tape behind affected ear)

Menopause: Black Moonstone, Blue Euclase, Eclipse Stone, Lodolite, Menalite, Peach Selenite

Mental:

abuse: Apricot Quartz, Lazurine, Proustite, Tugtupite with Nuummite, Yellow Crackle Quartz, Xenotine

agitation: Strawberry Quartz, Youngite

blockages: Molybdenite, Rhodozite

breakdown: Molybdenite, Novaculite, Quantum Quattro, Youngite. *Chakra:* third eye, crown

cleansing: Black Kyanite, Blue Quartz, Hungarian Quartz

clarity: Holly Agate, Merkabite Calcite, Moldau Quartz, Poldervaarite, Realgar and Orpiment, Sacred Scribe, Star Hollandite, Thompsonite

combine heart and mind: Adamite, Auralite 23

conditioning, rigid: Drusy Golden Healer, Pholocomite, Rainbow Covellite, and see Patterns pages 21, 54, 60, 97, 103, 137, 163. *Chakra:* third eye, crown

confusion: Aegerine, Blue Halite, Blue Quartz, Hematoid Calcite, Limonite, Pholocomite, Poldervaarite, Richterite

---

Unless otherwise directed, apply crystal over organ or site of symptom, place on appropriate chakra, wear as jewellery, bathe with or take as a crystal essence.

detox: Amechlorite, Banded Agate, Drusy Quartz on Sphalerite, Eye of the Storm, Larvikite, Pyrite in Magnesite, Rainbow Covellite, Smoky Quartz with Aegerine, Shungite, Richterite, Spirit Quartz, Tantalite

dexterity/flexibility, improve: Brucite, Bushman Quartz, Coprolite, Green Ridge Quartz, Kimberlite, Limonite, Molybdenite, Seriphos Quartz, Tiffany Stone, Titanite (Sphene). *Chakra:* third eye, crown

dysfunction: Alunite, Star Hollandite, Titanite (Sphene)

exhaustion: Cinnabar in Jasper, Marcasite, Spectrolite

focus: Sacred Scribe (Russian Lemurian)

implants: Amechlorite, Blue Halite, Brandenberg Amethyst, Cryolite, Drusy Golden Healer, Holly Agate, Ilmenite, Lemurian Aquitane Calcite, Novaculite, Nuummite, Pholocomite, Tantalite

sabotage: Agrellite, Amphibole, Lemurian Aquitane Calcite, Mohawkite, Paraiba Tourmaline, Yellow Scapolite, Tantalite

strength: Plancheite

undue influence, remove: Limonite, Novaculite, Tantalite

upheaval: Guinea Fowl Jasper

Menstruation: Menalite, Tugtupite

irregular: Menalite, Tugtupite. *Chakra:* sacral, base

Menstrual:

Unless otherwise directed, apply crystal over organ or site of symptom, place on appropriate chakra, wear as jewellery, bathe with or take as a crystal essence.

cramps: Bastnasite, Cat's Eye Quartz, Eilat Stone, Menalite, Orange Moss Agate, Serpentine in Obsidian, Shiva Lingam, Tugtupite. *Chakra:* sacral, base

cycle, regulate: Menalite, Tugtupite. *Chakra:* sacral, base

Mercury toxicity: see Heavy metals page 120

Meridians:

blocked: Apricot Quartz, Feather Pyrite, Orange Kyanite, Orange River, Polychrome Jasper, Pyrite in Quartz, Que Sera, Shiva Lingam, Snakeskin Pyrite, Spider Web Obsidian, Strawberry Lemurian. *Chakra:* dantien

harmonize planetary: Dragon Stone, Ethiopian Opal, Feather Pyrite, Mohawkite, Monazite, Polychrome Jasper, Que Sera, Spider Web Obsidian, Star Hollandite, Terraluminite

realign personal: Chrysotile in Serpentine, Feather Pyrite, Lemurian Seed, Polychrome Jasper, Orange River Quartz, Pink Lazurine, Terraluminite. *Chakra:* dantien

stimulate: Pyrite in Magnesite, Pyrite in Quartz, Que Sera, Shiva Lingam, Spider Web Obsidian. *Chakra:* dantien

Metabolism: *Chakra:* dantien

of fat: Pyrite in Magnesite

stimulate: Garnet in Pyroxene, Hackmanite, Pyrite in Magnesite, Tugtupite. *Chakra:* dantien, higher heart

---

Unless otherwise directed, apply crystal over organ or site of symptom, place on appropriate chakra, wear as jewellery, bathe with or take as a crystal essence.

regulate: Pearl Spa Dolomite

Metabolic:

imbalances: Amechlorite, Bornite, Champagne Aura Quartz, Galaxyite, Hackmanite, Khutnohorite, Sonora Sunrise, Tantalite, Tanzine Aura Quartz, Tugtupite, Winchite. *Chakra:* dantien, third eye

stimulating processes: Smoky Amethyst, Tugtupite. *Chakra:* dantien, third eye

syndrome: Anandalite, Andara Glass, Golden Azeztulite, Golden Danburite, Golden Herkimer, Healers Gold, Lemurian Jade, Mangano Vesuvianite, Quantum Quattro, Que Sera, Tanzine Aura Quartz

system: Amechlorite, Champagne Aura Quartz, Hackmanite, Piemontite, Smoky Amethyst, Smoky Quartz with Aegerine, Tantalite, Winchite

Miasms: Golden Danburite, Nuummite, Quantum Quattro. *Chakra:* earth star, base, past life

Microwaves: Shungite

Mid-life crisis: Bumble Bee Jasper, Eclipse Stone, Eklogite, Eye of the Storm

Migraine: Adularia, Afghanite, Cavansite, Gaia Stone, Herderite, Lazulite, Quantum Quattro, Pyrite in Magnesite, Rhodozite, Riebekite with Sugilite and Bustamite. *Chakra:* third eye, crown, past life

Mind: and see Mental page 144. *Chakra:* third eye, crown

Butterfly: Tantalite

chatter, switch off: Auralite 23, Bytownite,

Rhodozite, Rhomboid Selenite, Richterite, Scheelite and see Over-thinking page 158

control: Cryolite, Drusy Golden Healer, Pholocomite, Thunder Egg

malicious thoughts, release: Hemimorphite, Pholocomite, Scolecite

negative thought patterns: Amphibole, Arfvedsonite, Celadonite, Dumortierite, Nuummite, Owyhee Blue Opal, Rainbow Covellite, Scheelite, Scolecite

Minerals:

non-assimilation: Piemontite, Tantalite, Tanzine Aura Quartz

Miscarriage, healing after: Menalite. *Chakra:* sacral

Misfit: Tremolite. *Chakra:* base, dantien

Moles: Flint, Marcasite

Misogyny: Zircon

Mobility: Heulandite, Petrified Wood and see Joints page 131

Mood swings: Halite, Hanksite, Tantalite, Titanite (Sphene). *Chakra:* solar plexus

Motion sickness: Aztee, Gaspeite

Motor dysfunction: Axinite, Basalt, Bustamite, Cat's Eye Quartz, Cumberlandite, Golden Danburite, Klinoptilolith, Peanut Wood, Quartz with Epidote, Scolecite and Natrolite

Motor nerves: Bustamite, Cat's Eye Quartz, Golden Coracalcite, Scheelite

---

Unless otherwise directed, apply crystal over organ or site of symptom, place on appropriate chakra, wear as jewellery, bathe with or take as a crystal essence.

Mouth: Covellite

ulcers: Hemimorphite, Montebrasite

Mucus membranes: Conichalcite, Hanksite, Oregon Opal, Richterite

Multidimensional:

cellular healing: Ajo Blue Calcite, Ajo Quartz, Anandalite™, Annabergite, Brandenberg Amethyst, Crystal Cap Amethyst, Elestial Quartz, Eudialyte, Fire and Ice Quartz, Fiskenaesset Ruby, Golden Coracalcite, Golden Healer Quartz, Mangano Vesuvianite, Messina Quartz, Pollucite, Que Sera, Rhodozite, Ruby Lavender Quartz

connections: Ajoite, Anandalite™, Angelinite, Astraline, Azotic Topaz, Brandenberg Amethyst, Crystal Cap Amethyst, Crystalline Kyanite, Galaxyite, Hemimorphite, Lemurian Seed, Merlinite, Molybdenite in Quartz, Mystic Topaz, Natrolite, Nirvana Quartz, Sanda Rosa Azeztulite, Satyamani and Satyaloka Quartz, Spirit Quartz, Stellar Beam Calcite, Tiffany Stone

healing: Ajo Quartz, Anandalite™, Banded Agate, Celestobarite, Eudialyte, Fiskenaesset Ruby, Halite, Hanksite, Icicle Calcite, Kakortokite, Lilac Quartz, Lemurian Seed, Phantom Quartz, Que Sera, Rutile with Hematite, Sanda Rosa Azeztulite, Satyamani and Satyaloka Quartz, Shaman Quartz, Sichuan Quartz, Spirit Quartz, Tangerine Dream Lemurian, Trigonic

---

Unless otherwise directed, apply crystal over organ or site of symptom, place on appropriate chakra, wear as jewellery, bathe with or take as a crystal essence.

Quartz

self: Crystal Cap Amethyst, Herderite, Natrolite, Trigonic Quartz

soul work: Anandalite™, Brandenberg Amethyst, Fenster Quartz, Porphyrite (Chinese Letter Stone), Sugar Blade Quartz, Tanzine Aura Quartz, Trigonic Quartz

travel: Afghanite, Anandalite™, Auralite 23, Aztee, Banded Agate, Blue Moonstone, Brandenberg Amethyst, Celestobarite, Golden Selenite, Kinoite, Novaculite, Orange Creedite, Owyhee Blue Opal, Phantom Quartz, Polychrome Jasper, Preseli Bluestone, Rainbow Moonstone, Nunderite, Shaman Quartz, Spectrolite, Spirit Quartz, Sedona Stone, Tanzanite, Thunder Egg, Titanite (Sphene), Trigonic Quartz, Ussingite, Vivianite, Youngite

Multiple sclerosis: Angels Wing Calcite, Chrysotile, Chrysotile in Serpentine, Eudialyte, Scolecite and Natrolite. *Chakra:* dantien

Multiple personality disorder: Bastnasite, Brucite

Muscles: Bismuth, Black Kyanite, Cat's Eye Quartz, Petrified Wood, Nzuri Moyo, Phlogopite, Scheelite, Titanite (Sphene)

cramps: Bastnasite, Cat's Eye Quartz, Orange Moss Agate, Quantum Quattro, Serpentine in Obsidian, Strontianite and see page 92

flexibility: Cumberlandite, Kimberlite, Rosophia

---

pain: Aegirine, Blue Euclase, Cathedral Quartz, Eilat Stone, Flint, Rhodozite, Wind Fossil Agate

spasm: Bornite, Diopside, Malacholla, Phlogopite, Pyrite in Magnesite, Strontianite and see spasm page 187

strengthen: Aegirine, Bismuth, Bustamite

swelling: Anandalite™, Andean Blue Opal, Blue Euclase, Brochantite

tension: Basalt, Blue Aragonite, Blue Euclase, Champagne Aura Quartz

tissue: Desert Rose, Khutnohorite, Phlogopite, Sonora Sunrise

torn: Creedite, Diaspore (Zultanite), Nzuri Moyo, Tantalite

Muscular:

disorders: Diopside, Rosophia

dystrophy: Rosophia, Scolecite and Natrolite

Musculoskeletal system inflexibility: Coprolite, Kimberlite, Limonite, Quantum Quattro, Steatite, Stromatolite

- N -

Nails, strengthen: Bustamite, Pink Spa Dolomite, Riebekite with Sugilite and Bustamite

Narrow-mindedness: Kundalini Quartz. *Chakra:* base, higher heart

Nausea: Dumortierite, Gaspeite, Quantum Quattro. *Chakra:* solar plexus

Navel/sacral chakra: see Chakras page 76

Necessary change, accept: Axinite, Eclipse Stone, Ethiopian Opal, Luxullianite, Nunderite, Snakeskin Pyrite. *Chakra:* dantien

Neck: Blue Siberian Quartz. *Chakra:* throat

> **tension:** Alexandrite, Blue Moonstone, Blue Siberian Quartz, Rainbow Moonstone

Negative:

> **energy, dispel:** Black Kyanite, Guardian Stone, Hypersthene, Klinoptilolith, Nuummite, Smoky Elestial Quartz, Smoky Herkimer, Tantalite. *Chakra:* throat, earth star

> **karma:** Smoky Elestial Quartz and see Past life page 160. *Chakra:* past life

Negativity, dispel: Nuummite, Smoky Elestial Quartz, Tantalite. *Chakra:* earth star

Nerves: Bronzite, Cat's Eye Quartz, Cryolite, Dalmatian Stone, Golden Coracalcite, Merlinite, Nuummite, Phlogopite, Scheelite, Smoky Amethyst, Stichtite,

Tanzanite

calming: Eudialyte, Jamesonite

endings: Guinea Fowl Jasper, Tinguaite

motor: Bustamite, Cat's Eye Quartz

optic: see Eyes page 108

pain relief: Blue Euclase, Flint, Nuummite, Rhodozite, Wind Fossil Agate

regenerating: Natrolite with Scolecite

spinal: Tinguaite

strengthen: Banded Agate, Drusy Quartz on Sphalerite, Mystic Topaz, Nuummite

Nervous:

autonomic system: Anglesite, Barite, Datolite, Dendritic Chalcedony, Kambaba Jasper, Merlinite, Stichtite, Stromatolite, White Heulandite. *Chakra:* dantien

disorders: Natrolite with Scolecite

exhaustion: Cinnabar in Jasper, Eudialyte

stress: Eye of the Storm, Eudialyte, Larvikite, Merlinite, Riebekite with Sugilite and Bustamite, Shungite

sympathetic: Cumberlandite. *Chakra:* dantien

system: Aegirine, Alexandrite, Anglesite, Astrophyllite, Azeztulite with Morganite, Banded Agate, Datolite, Dendritic Chalcedony, Epidote, Eudialyte, Greenlandite, Kakortokite, Merlinite, Natrolite, Petrified Wood, Prehnite with Epidote,

Stichtite, Stichtite and Serpentine, White Heulandite
tension: Larvikite, Merlinite

Nervousness: Eudialyte

Neural fibres: Feather Pyrite, Pyrite and Sphalerite, Scolecite. *Chakra:* dantien

Neuralgia: Cat's Eye Quartz, Pyrite and Sphalerite

Neuritis: see Kidneys page 134

Neurological tissue: Alexandrite, Golden Coracalcite, Phlogopite, Scolecite and see Nerves above

Neurosis: Greenlandite. *Chakra:* solar plexus

Neurotic patterns: Arfvedsonite, Celadonite, Greenlandite, Porphyrite (Chinese Letter Stone), Rainbow Covellite, Scheelite. *Chakra:* solar plexus

Neurotransmitters: Anglesite, Crystal Cap Amethyst, Golden Coracalcite, Kambaba Jasper, Khutnohorite, Ocean Blue Jasper, Phantom Calcite, Que Sera, Scolecite, Shungite, Stromatolite, Tremolite. *Chakra:* alta major (base of skull)

Nervous system: Anglesite, Golden Coracalcite, Phantom Calcite

Neural pathways: Golden Coracalcite, Mystic Merlinite, Larvikite, Scolecite, Stichtite, Phantom Calcite

Nightmares/night terrors: Dalmatian Stone, Diaspore, Pearl Spa Dolomite, Spirit Quartz, Tremolite

Night:

  blindness: Blue Chalcedony, Golden Herkimer, Morion, Quantum Quattro, Sichuan Quartz, Tanzine

Aura Quartz, Vivianite

cramps/twitches: Blue or White Aragonite, Cat's Eye Quartz, Orange Moss Agate, Pearl Spa Dolomite, Serpentine in Obsidian

sweats: Blue Quartz, Indicolite Quartz, Menalite

terrors: Diaspore, Pearl Spa Dolomite, Smoky Amethyst, Smoky Elestial Quartz, Tremolite

NLP: Septarian

Nose: Covellite, Eclipse Stone, Goethite

   bleed: Hausmanite

Nuclear sites, neutralize radiation effects: Covellite, Hackmanite, Morion, Rainbow Covellite, Smoky Elestial Quartz, Tantalite, Torbernite, Velvet Malachite

Nutrient malabsorption: Blue Moonstone, Candle Quartz. *Chakra:* solar plexus

Nurturing, lack of: Amblygonite, Bornite on Silver, Calcite Fairy Stone, Clevelandite, Cobalto Calcite, Drusy Blue Quartz, Flint, Lazurine, Menalite, Mount Shasta Opal, Ocean Jasper, Prasiolite, Ruby Lavender Quartz, Septarian, Super 7, Tree Agate, Tugtupite. *Chakra:* higher heart, base

---

- O -

Obesity: Cassiterite, Epidote, Petrified Wood. *Chakra:* dantien

Obsession: Ammolite, Auralite 23, Barite, Bytownite, Fenster Quartz, Golden Selenite, Novaculite, Ocean Jasper, Red Amethyst, Spirit Quartz, Tantalite, Vera Cruz Amethyst. *Chakra:* dantien, solar plexus, third eye

Obsessive behaviour: Ocean Jasper, Smoky Rose Quartz, Tantalite

Obsessive-compulsive disorder: Amethyst Herkimer, Fenster Quartz, Flint, Novaculite, Tantalite

Obsessive thoughts: Ammolite, Auralite 23, Barite, Bytownite, Scolecite, Spirit Quartz, Tantalite. *Chakra:* third eye, crown

Odour absorption: Halite

Oesophagus: Indicolite Quartz, Goethite, Stibnite. *Chakra:* throat

Old age, overcome weakness in: Chrome Diopside, Flint, Kambaba Jasper, Schalenblende, Stromatolite. *Chakra:* dantien

Optic nerve: see Eyes page 108

Oppression: Blizzard Stone

Optimum functioning: Golden Healer Quartz

Osteoarthritis: Aztee, Brochantite, Calcite Fairy Stone, Chalcopyrite, Shungite, Tiffany Stone

Osteomyelitis: Ammolite

Unless otherwise directed, apply crystal over organ or site of symptom, place on appropriate chakra, wear as jewellery, bathe with or take as a crystal essence.

Osteoporosis: Morion Quartz, Wind Fossil Agate, Trummer Jasper

Osteitis: Ammolite

Outworn patterns: Amphibole, Arfvedsonite, Brandenberg Amethyst, Celadonite, Garnet in Quartz, Quantum Quattro, Owyhee Blue Opal, Porphyrite (Chinese Letter Stone), Rainbow Covellite, Rainbow Mayanite, Scheelite, Stibnite. *Chakra:* earth star, base, sacral, solar plexus, third eye

Ovaries: Menalite, Ocean Jasper, Schalenblende. *Chakra:* sacral

Ovulation pain: Blue Euclase, Crystalline Kyanite, Quantum Quattro, Rhodozite

Over:

  acidity: Agrellite, Bornite, Kimberlite, Klinoptilolith, Pyrophyllite

  active: Poppy Jasper

  alkalinity: Agrellite, Brucite, Gabbro

  attachment: Drusy Golden Healer, Rainbow Mayanite, Tantalite, Tinguaite. *Chakra:* solar plexus

  defended: Honey Opal

  dependent: Ussingite

  eating: Crystal Cap Amethyst, Epidote. *Chakra:* base, dantien

  excitability: Dumortierite, Fiskenaesset Ruby

  load: Diopside

  reaction: Paraiba Tourmaline

Unless otherwise directed, apply crystal over organ or site of symptom, place on appropriate chakra, wear as jewellery, bathe with or take as a crystal essence.

sensitive: Paraiba Tourmaline, Proustite, Riebekite with Sugilite and Bustamite, Scolecite, Shungite, Tremolite. *Chakra:* solar plexus

stimulated: Poppy Jasper

thinking: Auralite 23, Bytownite, Creedite, Dalmatian Stone, Rhomboid Selenite. *Chakra:* third eye

weight: Epidote, Ethiopian Opal, Hemimorphite, Heulandite, Petrified Wood

whelm: Diopside. *Chakra:* solar plexus

work: Prehnite with Epidote, Tanzanite

Oversensitive personality: Bastnasite, Hackmanite

Oversensitivity to:

cold: Barite

pressure: Avalonite

temperature changes: Barite, Dinosaur Bone, Luxullianite

weather: Avalonite, Barite, Golden Pietersite

Oxygen, malabsorption: Azotic Topaz, Banded Agate, Chinese Red Quartz, Goethite, Kambaba Jasper, Merlinite, Molybdenite, Pyrite in Magnesite, Pyrite in Quartz, Reinerite, Sonora Sunrise, Stromatolite. *Chakra:* dantien (or place over heart and lungs)

- P -

Pain relief: Bastnasite, Bird's Eye Jasper, Blue Euclase, Bronzite, Cathedral Quartz, Flint, Hungarian Quartz, Khutnohorite, Reinerite, Rhodozite, Stichtite and Serpentine, Wind Fossil Agate

Painful feelings, assimilate: Khutnohorite, Tugtupite. *Chakra:* heart

Palpitations: Dumortierite, Eye of the Storm, Honey Calcite. *Chakra:* dantien

Pancreas: Astraline, Bustamite, Brochantite, Chinese Chromium Quartz, Huebnerite, Leopardskin Jasper, Maw Sit Sit, Pink Opal, Quantum Quattro, Richterite, Schalenblende, Serpentine in Obsidian, Shungite, Tanzine Aura Quartz, Tugtupite. *Chakra:* spleen, dantien

Paradox, solve: Sulphur in Quartz

Paralysis: Petrified Wood

Pancreatic secretions: Astraline, Bustamite and see Blood sugar page 67 and Pancreas above. *Chakra:* spleen, solar plexus, base

Panic attacks: Dumortierite, Girasol, Green Phantom Quartz, Serpentine in Obsidian, Tremolite. *Chakra:* heart, solar plexus (keep in pocket and hold when required)

Parasites: Covellite, Cryolite, Proustite, Rainbow Covellite, Scolecite, Serpentine in Obsidian, Shungite, Smoky Amethyst (take as crystal essence and place over site of infestation)

Unless otherwise directed, apply crystal over organ or site of symptom, place on appropriate chakra, wear as jewellery, bathe with or take as a crystal essence.

Parathyroid: Blue Siberian Quartz, Cacoxenite, Champagne Aura Quartz, Chrysotile, Chrysotile in Serpentine, Cumberlandite, Leopardskin Jasper, Richterite, Tanzine Aura Quartz. *Chakra:* throat

Parkinson's disease: Anthrophyllite, Black Moonstone, Diaspore, Eudialyte, Kambaba Jasper, Owyhee Blue Opal, Nuummite, Stichtite, Stichtite and Serpentine, Stromatolite. *Chakra:* dantien

Past, release from: Dumortierite, Elestial Quartz, Smoky Amethyst and see Past life below. *Chakra:* past life, earth star, base

Past life: Brandenberg Amethyst, Nuummite, Oregon Opal, Rhodozite, Trigonic Quartz, Violane

> **abandonment:** Tugtupite. *Chakra:* past life, heart
>
> **access:** Brandenberg Amethyst, Cavansite, Dream Quartz, Dumortierite, Faden Quartz, Fiskenaesset Ruby, Lemurian Seed, Nuummite, Oregon Opal, Preseli Bluestone, Trigonic Quartz. *Chakra:* past life, third eye
>
> **addiction, causes of:** Crystal Cap Amethyst, Fenster Quartz, Kornerupine, Red Amethyst, Smoky Amethyst, Vera Cruz Amethyst. *Chakra:* past life, base
>
> **Akashic Record:** Afghanite, Amphibole, Andescine Labradorite, Blue Euclase, Brandenberg Amethyst, Brookite, Cathedral Quartz, Celestial Quartz, Chinese Writing Quartz, Dumortierite, Eilat Stone, Heulandite, Keyiapo, Lemurian Aquitane Calcite, Merkabite

---

Unless otherwise directed, apply crystal over organ or site of symptom, place on appropriate chakra, wear as jewellery, bathe with or take as a crystal essence.

Calcite, Merlinite, Phosphosiderite, Prophecy Stone, Serpentine in Obsidian, Sichuan Quartz, Tanzanite, Tremolite, Trigonic Quartz. *Chakra:* past life, third eye, crown

betrayal: Golden Green Ridge Quartz. *Chakra:* past life, heart

blockages from past lives: Ajo Blue Calcite, Lemurian Seed, Nuummite, Orange Kyanite, Purple Scapolite, Rainbow Mayanite, Rhodozite, Serpentine in Obsidian. *Chakra:* past life

break patterns: Arfvedsonite, Celadonite, Garnet in Quartz, Green Ridge Quartz, Lemurian Seed, Owyhee Blue Opal, Porphyrite (Chinese Letter Stone), Rainbow Covellite, Rainbow Mayanite, Rhodozite, Scheelite, Stellar Beam Calcite

broken heart: Cobalto Calcite, Mangano Vesuvianite, Tugtupite. *Chakra:* past life, heart

chastity, previous vow of: Kundalini Quartz, Menalite, Smoky Citrine. *Chakra*: past life, base, sacral

conflict: Bixbite, Champagne Aura Quartz, Fluorapatite, Purpurite, Rainbow Mayanite, Trigonic Quartz

contracts: Boli Stone, Dumortierite, Gabbro, Nuummite, Prasiolite, Purple Scapolite, Quantum Quattro, Red Amethyst

curses:

  break: Nuummite, Purpurite, Quantum Quattro,

Stibnite. *Chakra:* past life, throat, third eye

deflect effects of: Green Ridge Quartz, Quantum Quattro. *Chakra:* past life, throat

cycles: Fenster Quartz. *Chakra:* past life

death, unhealed trauma: Blue Euclase, Brandenberg Amethyst, Cavansite, Gaia Stone, Green Ridge Quartz, Lemurian Seed, Lemurian Jade, Oceanite, Quantum Quattro, Sea Sediment Jasper, Smoky Elestial Quartz, Spirit Quartz, Tantalite, Victorite. *Chakra:* past life, earth star, base, heart

debts, recognize: Lemurian Seed, Nuummite, Purple Scapolite. *Chakra:* past life, solar plexus

dis-ease: Dumortierite, Lemurian Seed, Sichuan Quartz. *Chakra:* past life

effects on present: Rhodozite

emotional:

   attachments: Aegirine, Drusy Golden Healer, Ilmenite, Novaculite, Nuummite, Rainbow Mayanite, Smoky Amethyst, Stibnite, Tantalite, Tinguaite. *Chakra:* past life

   body: Oregon Opal

   healing: Cobalto Calcite, Boli Stone, Mangano Vesuvianite

   hooks: Drusy Golden Healer, Goethite, Nunderite, Orange Kyanite, Pyromorphite, Tantalite

   pain: Blue Euclase, Cobalto Calcite. *Chakra:* past life, heart, higher heart, solar plexus

planning: Stellar Beam Calcite

trauma: Ajo Blue Calcite, Blue Euclase, Cavansite, Gaia Stone, Guinea Fowl Jasper, Holly Agate, Mangano Vesuvianite, Oceanite, Oregon Opal, Peanut Wood, Ruby Lavender Quartz, Sea Sediment Jasper, Tantalite, Victorite

wounds: Ajo Quartz, Eudialyte, Fiskenaesset Ruby, Macedonian Opal, Moldau Quartz, Mookaite Jasper, Prehnite with Epidote, Rathbunite™, Rosophia, Scheelite, Tangerose, Tugtupite, Xenotine. *Chakra:* past life, heart, higher heart, solar plexus

entity attachment: Chrysotile in Serpentine, Drusy Golden Healer, Ilmenite, Larvikite, Lemurian Aquitane Calcite, Novaculite, Nuummite, Pyromorphite, Quantum Quattro, Rainbow Mayanite, Stibnite, Tantalite, Tinguaite, Tugtupite, Valentinite and Stibnite. *Chakra:* past life, sacral, solar plexus, spleen, third eye

family patterns: Arfvedsonite, Brandenberg Amethyst, Celadonite, Fenster Quartz, Dumortierite, Garnet in Quartz, Polychrome Jasper, Porphyrite (Chinese Letter Stone), Rainbow Covellite, Scheelite. *Chakra:* past life, sacral

grief, unhealed: Empowerite, Mangano Vesuvianite, Oregon Opal, Tugtupite, Voegesite. *Chakra:* past life, heart

---

Unless otherwise directed, apply crystal over organ or site of symptom, place on appropriate chakra, wear as jewellery, bathe with or take as a crystal essence.

healing: Blizzard Stone, Chinese Red Quartz, Dumortierite, Garnet in Quartz, Lodolite, Oregon Opal, Picasso Jasper, Peanut Wood, Serpentine in Obsidian, Tanzanite, Tibetan Quartz, Tugtupite, Voegesite. *Chakra:* past life

heart pain/heartbreak: Blue Euclase, Brandenberg Amethyst, Cobalto Calcite, Mangano Vesuvianite, Tugtupite. *Chakra:* past life, higher heart

hyperactivity due to effects of: Dianite, Yellow Scapolite. *Chakra:* past life, third eye

imperatives: Ammolite, Lemurian Aquitane Calcite, Novaculite, Tantalite

implants: Amechlorite, Cryolite, Drusy Golden Healer, Holly Agate, Ilmenite, Lemurian Aquitane Calcite, Novaculite, Nuummite, Rainbow Mayanite, Tantalite, Tinguaite

injuries: Flint. *Chakra:* past life

jealousies: Rainbow Mayanite

learning from: Dumortierite. *Chakra:* past life

manipulation: Nuummite, Tantalite

memories: Dream Quartz

mental imperatives, release: Golden Danburite, Nuummite, Septarian, Tantalite. *Chakra:* past life

misuse of power: Ocean Jasper, Nuummite, Smoky Lemurian Seed

phobias resulting from: Carolite, Dumortierite, Oceanite, Serpentine in Obsidian. *Chakra:* past life

Unless otherwise directed, apply crystal over organ or site of symptom, place on appropriate chakra, wear as jewellery, bathe with or take as a crystal essence.

pollutants: Diaspore (Zultanite), Paraiba Tourmaline, Phlogopite, Pyrite and Sphalerite, Pyromorphite, Shungite

psychosexual problems resulting from: Cobalto Calcite, Dumortierite, Serpentine in Obsidian. *Chakra:* past life, base, sacral

recall: Dumortierite, Preseli Bluestone, Revelation Stone. *Chakra:* past life, third eye

reclaim power: Brandenberg Amethyst, Eilat Stone, Empowerite, Leopardskin Jasper, Nuummite, Owyhee Blue Opal, Rainbow Mayanite, Smoky Elestial Quartz, Tinguaite. *Chakra:* past life, base

regression: Dumortierite, Preseli Bluestone, Wind Fossil Agate. *Chakra:* past life, third eye

relationships: Smoky Amethyst. *Chakra:* past life, base, sacral, heart

releasing vows: Nuummite, Rainbow Mayanite, Stibnite, Wind Fossil Agate. *Chakra:* past life, third eye

rejection: Cassiterite. *Chakra:* past life, heart

resentment: Eclipse Stone, Tugtupite. *Chakra:* past life, base

restraint, psychological, emotional or mental: Libyan Gold Tektite, Tugtupite. *Chakra:* past life, heart

sexual problems arising from: Eilat Stone, Rutile. *Chakra:* past life, base, sacral

soul agreements, recognition: Brandenberg Amethyst, Green Ridge Quartz, Nuummite, Trigonic

Quartz, Wind Fossil Agate. *Chakra:* past life, higher crown

soul loss resulting from: Chrysotile in Serpentine, Fulgarite

tie cutting: Flint, Novaculite, Nuummite, Rainbow Mayanite, Smoky Amethyst. *Chakra:* past life, base, sacral, solar plexus, third eye

thought forms, release: Aegirine, Pyromorphite, Scolecite, Septarian, Spectrolite, Xenotine. *Chakra:* past life, third eye

trauma: Blue Euclase, Brandenberg Amethyst, Dumortierite, Empowerite, Mangano Vesuvianite, Oceanite, Oregon Opal, Smoky Elestial Quartz, Red Phantom Quartz, Ruby Lavender Quartz, Smoky Herkimer, Tantalite, Victorite

vows, release: Andean Opal, Dumortierite, Libyan Gold Tektite, Nuummite, Rainbow Mayanite. *Chakra:* past life

wound imprints in etheric body: Ajo Quartz, Brandenberg Amethyst, Diaspore (Zultanite), Ethiopian Opal, Eye of the Storm, Flint, Green Ridge Quartz, Lemurian Aquitane Calcite, Lemurian Seed, Macedonian Opal, Master Shamanite, Mookaite Jasper, Rainbow Mayanite, Snakeskin Pyrite, Stibnite, Tantalite. *Chakra:* past life or place over site

People-pleaser: Anthrophyllite. *Chakra:* dantien

Perception, sense: Schalenblende

Unless otherwise directed, apply crystal over organ or site of symptom, place on appropriate chakra, wear as jewellery, bathe with or take as a crystal essence.

Periodontal disease: White Drusy Quartz

Peripheral circulation: Dianite, Garnet in Quartz, Ouro Verde, Riebekite with Sugilite and Bustamite. *Chakra:* dantien

Period pains/PMS: Bastnasite, Beryllonite, Blue Euclase, Lodolite, Menalite, Orange Kyanite, Quantum Quattro, Rhodozite, Serpentine in Obsidian. *Chakra:* sacral

Personal growth: Axinite

Personal power:

    increase: Basalt, Brandenberg Amethyst, Conichalcite, Empowerite, Eudialyte, Eye of the Storm, Orange Kyanite, Owyhee Blue Opal, Sedona Stone, Shungite, Tinguaite. *Chakra:* base, dantien

    overcome misuse of: Nuummite, Smoky Lemurian. *Chakra:* past life, base

Personality disorders: use crystals under the guidance of a qualified crystal therapist

Pesticides: Shungite

pH balance: Rhodozite

Phobias: Andean Blue Opal, Dumortierite, Frondellite with Strengite, Girasol, Hackmanite, Oceanite. *Chakra:* past life, solar plexus, base

Physical:

    body, discomfort at being in: Empowerite, Larvikite, Pearl Spa Dolomite, Strontianite. *Chakra:* earth star, base, dantien, soma

    endurance, improve: Poppy Jasper, Schalenblende.

Unless otherwise directed, apply crystal over organ or site of symptom, place on appropriate chakra, wear as jewellery, bathe with or take as a crystal essence.

Chakra: earth star, base, dantien

exhaustion: Mariposite, Judy's Jasper, Poppy Jasper, Purpurite, Red Lemurian Seed Crystal. *Chakra:* earth star, base, dantien

pleasure, share: Poppy Jasper. *Chakra:* earth star, base

weakness: Diopside, Schalenblende, Sedona Stone. *Chakra:* dantien

well-being: Cloudy Quartz, Golden Healer Quartz, Guardian Stone, Keyiapo, Quantum Quattro, Que Sera, Schalenblende, Sedona Stone, Shungite. *Chakra:* earth star, base, dantien

Pineal gland: Blue Moonstone, Champagne Aura Quartz, Fire and Ice Quartz, Fluorapatite, Preseli Bluestone, Richterite, Tanzine Aura Quartz, Tanzanite, Tremolite. *Chakra:* third eye

Pituitary gland: Champagne Aura Quartz, Fire and Ice Quartz, Tanzine Aura Quartz. *Chakra:* third eye

Plague, ward off: Shungite

Planetary realignment: Cacoxenite, Eye of the Storm

Plans, bring to fruition: Chinese Writing Stone

PMS: see Period pains page 167

Pneumonia: Shungite (drink two litres Shungite water daily), Tanzine Aura Quartz

Pollen allergies: Bastnasite, Bumble Bee Jasper, Ouro Verde, Shungite

Pollutants, anti: Champagne Aura Quartz, Diaspore (Zultanite), Nuummite, Phlogopite, Pyrite and

---

Unless otherwise directed, apply crystal over organ or site of symptom, place on appropriate chakra, wear as jewellery, bathe with or take as a crystal essence.

Sphalerite, Pyromorphite, Shungite, Smoky Elestial Quartz. *Chakra:* earth star

Pomposity: Turritella Agate

'Poor me' syndrome: Lemurian Jade

Post-natal depression: Ajo Blue Calcite, Rainbow Goethite, Sillimanite. *Chakra:* solar plexus, sacral

Post-operative recovery: Empowerite, Eye of the Storm, Fire Obsidian, Marialite, Petrified Wood, Prehnite with Epidote, Scapolite, Stromatolite. *Chakra:* dantien

Post Traumatic Stress disorder: Bird's Eye Jasper, Eisenkiesel, Empowerite, Eye of the Storm, Richterite, Shungite, Tantalite, Victorite. *Chakra:* dantien, higher heart

Poverty consciousness: Citrine Herkimer, Smoky Citrine, Tugtupite. *Chakra:* sacral

Powerlessness: Basalt, Eye of the Storm, Nuummite, Smoky Elestial Quartz. *Chakra:* base, dantien

Pregnancy: Menalite. *Chakra:* sacral

    support during: Menalite

    fatigue during: Apricot Quartz

Premature ejaculation: Rutile

Pressure changes, sensitivity to: Avalonite

Pride: Cobalto Calcite. *Chakra:* heart

Procrastination: Montebrasite. *Chakra:* dantien

Problem, solve: Eilat Stone, Shaman Quartz with Rutile. *Chakra:* third eye

Projections: Spectrolite, Vivianite, Voegesite. *Chakra:*

Unless otherwise directed, apply crystal over organ or site of symptom, place on appropriate chakra, wear as jewellery, bathe with or take as a crystal essence.

third eye, solar plexus

Prolonged illness: see Chronic illness page 84

Prostate: Brochantite, Bustamite, Schalenblende. *Chakra:* base

    enlarged: Calcite Fairy Stone

Protection: Guinea Fowl Jasper, Lorenzenite (Ramsayite), Nunderite, Richterite, Tantalite, Master Shamanite. *Chakra:* throat, higher heart

Protein assimilation: see Assimilation page 56

Psoriasis: Conichalcite, Faden Quartz, Guinea Fowl Jasper, Snakeskin Agate, Wind Fossil Agate (bathe in crystal essence and apply stone to site)

Psychic:

    attack, protect against: Brandenburg Amethyst, Master Shamanite, Mohawkite, Nunderite, Nuummite, Polychrome Jasper, Richterite, Tantalite, Tugtupite. (Wear constantly.) *Chakra:* throat, higher heart

    blockages: Afghanite, Ajo Quartz, Bytownite, Blue Selenite, Rhodozite

    implants/imprints: Amechlorite, Brandenberg Amethyst, Cryolite, Drusy Golden Healer, Ethiopian Opal, Flint, Holly Agate, Ilmenite, Lemurian Aquitane Calcite, Novaculite, Nuummite, Pyromorphite, Rainbow Mayanite, Snakeskin Pyrite, Stichtite, Tantalite

    interference: Afghanite, Master Shamanite,

Nuummite, Purpurite, Rainbow Mayanite, Tantalite

manipulation: Nuummite

mugging: Tugtupite. *Chakra:* higher heart

overwhelm: Limonite, Master Shamanite

shield: Actinolite, Amphibole, Azotic Topaz, Aztee, Bornite, Bowenite (New Jade), Brandenberg Amethyst, Brazilianite, Celestobarite, Chlorite Shaman Quartz, Crackled Fire Agate, Fiskenaesset Ruby, Frondellite with Strengite, Gabbro, Graphic Smoky Quartz (Zebra Stone), Hanksite, Iridescent Pyrite, Keyiapo, Lorenzenite (Ramsayite), Marcasite, Mohave Turquoise, Master Shamanite, Mohawkite, Owyhee Blue Opal, Polychrome Jasper, Purpurite, Pyromorphite, Quantum Quattro, Red Amethyst, Silver Leaf Jasper, Smoky Amethyst, Smoky Elestial Quartz, Tantalite, Thunder Egg, Valentinite and Stibnite, Xenotine

surgery: Eisenkiesel, Flint, Lemurian Seed, Rainbow Mayanite Schalenblende, Seriphos Quartz

trauma: Blue Euclase, Empowerite, Lemurian Seed, Mangano Vesuvianite, Oceanite, Smoky Lemurian Seed, Morion, Ruby Lavender Quartz, Tangerine Aura Quartz, Tantalite, Victorite

vampirism: Ammolite, Apple Aura Quartz, Actinolite, Banded Agate, Gaspeite, Iridescent Pyrite, Lemurian Aquitane Calcite, Nunderite, Prasiolite, Tantalite, Xenotine

---

Unless otherwise directed, apply crystal over organ or site of symptom, place on appropriate chakra, wear as jewellery, bathe with or take as a crystal essence.

Psychological:

    autonomy: Pyrophyllite, Xenotine. *Chakra:* dantien

    balance: Amblygonite

    catharsis: Barite, Epidote, Gaia Stone, Nirvana Quartz, Smoky Elestial Quartz, Smoky Spirit Quartz

    healing: Agrellite, Ajoite, Annabergite, Black Kyanite, Diopside, Flint, Fulgarite, Lemurian Jade, Lemurian Seed, Nuummite, Ocean Jasper, Quantum Quattro, Smoky Elestial, Stellar Beam Calcite

    insights: Actinolite, Smoky Brandenberg Amethyst, Lazulite, Leopardskin Serpentine, Septarian, Shiva Lingam

    safety: Tree Agate, Xenotine

    shadow: Agrellite, Azeztulite with Morganite, Champagne Aura Quartz, Covellite, Day and Night Quartz, Lazulite, Lemurian Seed, Molybdenite, Nuummite, Phantom Quartz, Proustite, Shaman Quartz, Smoky Elestial Quartz, Voegesite. *Chakra:* solar plexus

    union: Graphic Smoky Quartz, Zebra Stone, Zircon

Psychosexual problems: Eilat Stone. *Chakra:* base, sacral

Psychosomatic disease: Andescine Labradorite, Angels Wing Calcite, Astraline, Azeztulite with Morganite, Azotic Topaz, Benitoite, Dumortierite, Fire Obsidian, Gaia Stone, Golden Danburite, Icicle Calcite, Larvikite, Ocean Blue Jasper, Roselite, Snakeskin Pyrite, Titanite (Sphene), Voegesite. *Chakra:* third eye, higher heart

---

Unless otherwise directed, apply crystal over organ or site of symptom, place on appropriate chakra, wear as jewellery, bathe with or take as a crystal essence.

sexual: Azeztulite with Morganite

stabilize body during changes: Basalt, Huebnerite, Luxullianite, Nunderite, Snakeskin Pyrite, Tangerose

understand causes of: Azotic Topaz, Benitoite, Chalcopyrite, Faden Quartz, Icicle Calcite, Kornerupine, Stichtite and Serpentine, Voegesite

Pollutants in atmosphere: Eye of the Storm, Hackmanite, Kambaba Jasper, Pyrite and Sphalerite, Pyromorphite, Shungite, Stromatolite

Pregnancy: Blue Euclase, Menalite

Puberty: Blue Euclase, Menalite, Peach Selenite

Public speaking: Owyhee Blue Opal, Septarian, Titanite (Sphene)

Pulmonary system: Indicolite Quartz and see Lungs page 141

Pulse, irregular: Ammolite, Cavansite, Creedite, Eye of the Storm, Serpentine in Obsidian. *Chakra:* dantien

Purification: Halite, Hanksite

Pus: Shungite

Pustules: Purpurite

Unless otherwise directed, apply crystal over organ or site of symptom, place on appropriate chakra, wear as jewellery, bathe with or take as a crystal essence.

- Q -

Qi: *Chakra:* sacral, dantien

    depleted: Ammolite, Budd Stone (African Jade), Chalcopyrite, Granite, Judy's Jasper, Poppy Jasper, Que Sera, Ruby in Granite, Rhodozite, Sonora Sunrise, Violane, Witches Finger

    transmit: Feather Pyrite, Que Sera, Rhodozite, Terraluminite

Quinsy: Chrysotile, Owyhee Blue Opal, Shungite (gargle with Shungite water). *Chakra:* throat

---

Unless otherwise directed, apply crystal over organ or site of symptom, place on appropriate chakra, wear as jewellery, bathe with or take as a crystal essence.

- R -

Racial conflict: see Ethnic conflict page 108

Racism: Catlinite, Zircon

Radiation, counteract: Covellite, Hackmanite, Klinoptilolith, Morion, Ouro Verde, Rainbow Covellite, Smoky Elestial, Tantalite, Torbernite, Uranophane, Velvet Malachite (under supervision). *Chakra:* earth star, base

Radionics: Agrellite, Blizzard Stone

Radiotherapy: Annabergite, Morion, Smoky Elestial Quartz, Tantalite, Torbernite (under supervision), Velvet Malachite

Radon gas: Diaspore, Ouro Verde, Morion Quartz, Smoky Elestial

Rashes: Cryolite, Snakeskin Agate

Raynaud's disease: Blue Aragonite, Dianite, Ouro Verde, Reinerite. *Chakra:* dantien

Rebirthing: Khutnohorite, Poppy Jasper, Smoky Amethyst, Spirit Quartz, Steatite, Voegesite. *Chakra:* sacral

Reconciliation: Afghanite, Chinese Red Quartz, Pink Lazurine, Ruby Lavender Quartz. *Chakra:* heart seed

Recovery, assist: Empowerite, Eye of the Storm, Fire Obsidian, Petrified Wood, Prehnite with Epidote, Quantum Quattro, Que Sera, Stromatolite. *Chakra:* dantien

---

Unless otherwise directed, apply crystal over organ or site of symptom, place on appropriate chakra, wear as jewellery, bathe with or take as a crystal essence.

Rectal disorders: Bastnasite

Recuperation: Poppy Jasper, Quantum Quattro, Que Sera. *Chakra:* dantien

Red blood cells: see Blood page 65

Reflexes: Dalmatian Stone

Reiki support: Andara Glass, Crackle Quartz, Pollucite, Shift Crystal, Stone of Sanctuary (place in room)

Rejection, ease pain of: Cassiterite, Tugtupite. *Chakra:* higher

Rejuvenation: Judy's Jasper, Menalite, Poppy Jasper. *Chakra:* dantien

Relaxation: Mystic Topaz. *Chakra:* third eye (hold or wear, place by bed)

Relationship:

    end gracefully: Eudialyte

    harmonize: Scolecite

    past sell-by date: Wind Fossil Agate

Release anger and tension: Alabaster, Blue Phantom Quartz, Chinese Red Quartz, Cinnabar in Jasper, Ethiopian Opal, Greenlandite, Nzuri Moyo, Pearl Spa Dolomite, Phosphosiderite, Tugtupite, Ussingite. *Chakra:* base, dantien

Renal disorders: see Kidneys page 134

Renewal: Ocean Jasper (tape over higher heart chakra)

Repair, assist body to: Aegirine, Bixbite, Brandenberg Amethyst, Celestial Quartz, Rutile with Hematite, Molybdenite. *Chakra:* dantien

---

Unless otherwise directed, apply crystal over organ or site of symptom, place on appropriate chakra, wear as jewellery, bathe with or take as a crystal essence.

Repetitive strain injury: Frondellite

Repressed:

    anger: Cinnabar in Jasper, Ethiopian Opal, Nzuri Moyo, Phosphosiderite. *Chakra:* base, dantien

    emotions: Ethiopian Opal

Reproductive system: Beryllonite, Black Kyanite, Calcite Fairy Stone, Fire and Ice Quartz, Lepidocrosite, Menalite, Voegesite, Xenotine. *Chakra:* base, sacral, dantien

    fallopian tubes: Menalite, Schalenblende. *Chakra:* sacral

    female: Black Moonstone, Fire and Ice Quartz, Menalite, Schalenblende, Tangerose. *Chakra:* sacral, base

    inflammation: Blue Euclase, Dendritic Chalcedony, Hanksite, Kundalini Quartz, Rhodozite, Sulphur in Quartz

    male: Calcite Fairy Stone, Schalenblende, Shiva Lingam

    ovaries: Menalite, Schalenblende

    testicles: Alexandrite, Schalenblende. *Chakra:* base

Rescind vows: Banded Agate, Brandenberg Amethyst, Dumortierite

Rescue essence: Quantum Quattro, Que Sera, Tangerose (take crystal essence frequently or apply stones)

Resentment: Eclipse Stone, Eudialyte. *Chakra:* base, dantien

Resistance to change: Dragon Stone, Eclipse Stone,

Unless otherwise directed, apply crystal over organ or site of symptom, place on appropriate chakra, wear as jewellery, bathe with or take as a crystal essence.

Luxullianite, Montebrasite, Snakeskin Pyrite, Tangerose. *Chakra*: base, dantien, heart

Respiratory system: Blue Aragonite, Cacoxenite, Halite, Merlinite, Prophecy Stone, Pyrite in Quartz, Richterite, Riebekite with Sugilite and Bustamite, Smoky Amethyst, Snakeskin Pyrite, Tremolite. *Chakra:* dantien, higher heart

    problems: Cacoxenite, Riebekite with Sugilite and Bustamite, Smoky Amethyst, Tremolite

Retrieval, child or soul parts: Fulgarite, Khutnohorite, Tangerose

Rheumatism: Granite

Rheumatoid arthritis: Aztee, Halite, Reinerite, Shungite

Rickets: Calcite Fairy Stone, Granite

RNA stabilizing: Chalcopyrite. *Chakra:* dantien

- S -

Sabotage: Lemurian Aquitane Calcite, Mohawkite, Scapolite, Scheelite
Sacral chakra: see Chakras page 76
Sadness: Indicolite Quartz. *Chakra:* solar plexus, heart
Safe passage: Flint, Gaspeite, Stibnite, Preseli Bluestone
Saviour complex: Cassiterite
Scalds: see Burns page 71
Scalp: Bowenite (New Jade)
Scapegoating behaviour: Champagne Aura Quartz, Mohawkite, Smoky Amethyst, Scapolite
Scar tissue: Khutnohorite, Tantalite
Sciatica: Zircon
Seasonal affective disorder: Adamite, Golden Selenite, Kakortokite, Pink Sunstone, Septarian, Sunshine Aura Quartz, Tugtupite. *Chakra:* third eye
Security issues: Chinese Red Quartz, Nzuri Moyo. *Chakra:* base
    emotional: Mangano Vesuvianite, Oceanite, Tugtupite. *Chakra:* base, dantien, solar plexus
    letting go of: Axinite, Scheelite. *Chakra:* base, dantien
Sedation: Poppy Jasper
Self:
    acceptance: Lavender Quartz, Lemurian Seed, Orange Phantom, Peach Selenite, Quantum Quattro, Tangerose, Tugtupite. *Chakra:* heart, higher heart

---

Unless otherwise directed, apply crystal over organ or site of symptom, place on appropriate chakra, wear as jewellery, bathe with or take as a crystal essence.

awareness: Citrine Spirit Quartz

confidence: Blue Quartz, Lemurian Seed, Nunderite, Pink Sunstone

criticism: Epidote

deception: Oregon Opal

defeating programs: Desert Rose, Drusy Quartz, Kinoite, Nuummite, Paraiba Tourmaline, Quantum Quattro, Strawberry Quartz

discipline: Blue Quartz, Dumortierite, Scapolite, Sillimanite

development: Hemimorphite

doubt: Rosophia

esteem: Eisenkiesel, Graphic Smoky Quartz (Zebra Stone), Hackmanite, Lazulite, Morion, Nzuri Moyo, Pink Phantom, Strawberry Quartz, Tinguaite. *Chakra:* base, sacral, dantien, heart, higher heart

expression: Eilat Stone, Mariposite, Owyhee Blue Opal. *Chakra:* throat

forgiveness: Chinese Red Quartz, Eudialyte, Pink Crackle Quartz, Spirit Quartz, Steatite, Tugtupite

hatred (combating): Blizzard Stone, Quantum Quattro, Tugtupite. *Chakra:* base

healing: Benitoite, Elestial Quartz, Eudialyte, Faden Quartz, Gaia Stone, Morion, Quantum Quattro, Rosophia, Septarian

image, poor: Dianite, Kinoite, Trummer Jasper

integrating: Ajoite, Amethyst Herkimer, Brandenberg

Amethyst, Eilat Stone, Faden Quartz, Quantum Quattro, Sichuan Quartz

nurturing: Poppy Jasper, Quantum Quattro, Septarian, Smoky Cathedral Quartz, Super 7

pity: Epidote

preservation: Dumortierite

respect: Rainforest Jasper

sabotaging behaviour: Agrellite, Quantum Quattro, Scapolite

sufficiency: Nunderite, Quantum Quattro. *Chakra:* base

trust: Honey Calcite. *Chakra:* sacral

worth: Rose Aura Quartz. *Chakra:* base, sacral

Senile dementia: Anthrophyllite, Stichtite and Serpentine. *Chakra:* third eye

Senior moments: Barite, Hematoid Calcite, Herderite, Marcasite, Vivianite

Sense of smell, loss: Fluorapatite, Schalenblende

Sensory organs, desensitized: Schalenblende. *Chakra:* dantien

Septicaemia: Quantum Quattro, Shungite

Severe illness: Diopside, Kambaba Jasper, Poppy Jasper, Quantum Quattro. *Chakra:* dantien

Sexual:

abuse, healing: Apricot Quartz, Azeztulite with Morganite, Eilat Stone, Honey Opal, Lazurine, Orange Kyanite, Pink Crackle Quartz, Proustite,

Shiva Lingam, Xenotine. *Chakra:* base, sacral, dantien

dysfunction: Orange Kyanite

libido, loss of: Orange Kyanite, Poppy Jasper, Shiva Lingam, Shungite. *Chakra:* base, sacral, dantien

organs: Menalite, Shiva Lingam. *Chakra:* base, sacral

pleasure, prolong: Poppy Jasper. *Chakra:* base, sacral

Shadow, integrate: Morion, Proustite, Smoky Lemurian Seed, Voegesite

Shame: Azeztulite with Morganite, Catlinite. *Chakra:* base, dantien

Shamanic journey: Brandenberg Amethyst, Celestobarite, Chrysotile in Serpentine, Graphic Smoky Quartz (Zebra Stone), Leopardskin Jasper, Lodolite, Mount Shasta Opal, Nunderite, Owyhee Blue Opal, Polychrome Jasper, Scolecite, Serpentine in Obsidian, Shaman Quartz, Smoky Quartz with Aegerine, Stibnite, Titanite (Sphene) see also Journeying page 132

Shape shifting: Leopardskin Jasper, Serpentine in Obsidian, Mount Shasta Opal. *Chakra:* soma/third eye

Shingles: Guinea Fowl Jasper, Silver Agate

Shock: Eye of the Storm (Judy's Jasper), Quantum Quattro, Que Sera, Richterite, Smoky Elestial Quartz, Tantalite. *Chakra:* solar plexus (take crystal essence frequently or wear stones constantly)

  Anaphylactic: Ouro Verde

Shoulders: Empowerite, Prehnite with Epidote, Scapolite

  frozen: Ice Quartz. *Chakra:* throat

Unless otherwise directed, apply crystal over organ or site of symptom, place on appropriate chakra, wear as jewellery, bathe with or take as a crystal essence.

psychosomatic reasons behind frozen: Gaia Stone, Prehnite with Epidote, Scapolite

Shyness: Barite, Owyhee Blue Opal (wear constantly)

Sick-building syndrome: Hackmanite, Morion, Smoky Elestial Quartz, Trummer Jasper (place around building, place zigzag in room see page 45, or wear constantly)

Side effects, drugs: Dogtooth Calcite

Sight: Cat's Eye Quartz, Vivianite and see Eyes page 108. *Chakra:* third eye

Sinuses: Brochantite, Champagne Aura Quartz, Covellite, Eilat Stone, Titanite (Sphene). *Chakra:* third eye

Sinusitis: Covellite, Indicolite Quartz, Titanite (Sphene) (place over nostrils or forehead, or inhale crystal essence steam)

Skeletal system: Coprolite, Crinoidal Limestone, Empowerite, Golden Coracalcite, Limonite, Pearl Spa Dolomite, Phantom Calcite, Poldervaarite, Pyromorphite, Steatite, Stromatolite, Turritella Agate, Tinguaite. *Chakra:* third eye

> **flexibility, improve:** Coprolite, Kimberlite, Tinguaite
>
> **support growth in youth:** Limonite

Skin: Bustamite, Chohua Jasper, Eisenkiesel, Epidote, Ethiopian Opal, Guinea Fowl Jasper, Halite, Hanksite, Honey Calcite, Kieseltuff, Klinoptilolith, Pearl Spa Dolomite, Phosphosiderite, Prehnite with Epidote, Riebekite with Sugilite and Bustamite, Snakeskin Agate, Stichtite, Titanite (Sphene)

Unless otherwise directed, apply crystal over organ or site of symptom, place on appropriate chakra, wear as jewellery, bathe with or take as a crystal essence.

ageing, reverse: Snakeskin Agate

cancer: Fluorapatite, Klinoptilolith (place over site)

detoxify: Aegirine, Amechlorite, Eye of the Storm, Graphic Smoky Quartz, Jamesonite, Larvikite, Pyrite in Magnesite, Richterite, Shungite, Smoky Elestial Quartz, Smoky Quartz with Aegerine, Rainbow Covellite, Stichtite

disorders: Erythrite, Leopardskin Jasper, Spirit Quartz

elasticity: Epidote, Flint, Novaculite, Stichtite

encrustations: Drusy Golden Healer, Faden Quartz, Prophecy Stone, Wind Fossil Agate

growths: Kieseltuff, Wind Fossil Agate

infections: Shungite

inflammation: Chrysotile in Serpentine, Guinea Fowl Jasper, Rhodozite, Sulphur in Quartz

stretch marks: Stichtite

Sleep: see Insomnia page 127

Sluggishness: Poppy Jasper, Quantum Quattro, Que Sera. *Chakra:* base, dantien

Smell, restore sense of: Fluorapatite

Smoking: Botswana Agate (wear constantly; dowse for underlying cause and treat accordingly)

giving up: Botswana Agate

Snakebite: Serpentine

Soft tissue damage: Diaspore (Zultanite), Eilat Stone, Eisenkiesel, Flint, Khutnohorite, Piemontite, Phlogopite,

Tantalite

Solar plexus chakra: see Chakras page 76

Soma chakra: see Chakras page 76

Sorcery: Nuummite, Purpurite

Sore throat: Shungite, Owyhee Blue Opal. *Chakra:* throat (gargle with crystal essence or wear stone at throat)

Sores: Shungite

Sorrow: Tugtupite. *Chakra:* heart

Soul: Brandenberg Amethyst, Cathedral Quartz, Golden Danburite, Nirvana Quartz, Trigonic Quartz. *Chakra:* higher crown, heart

   cleanser: Anandalite, Black Kyanite, Brandenberg Amethyst, Chinese Chromium Quartz, Chrysotile in Serpentine, Golden Danburite, Khutnohorite, Prehnite with Epidote, Rutile with Hematite, Smoky Cathedral Quartz, Smoky Elestial Quartz

   contracts, release: Black Kyanite, Boli Stone, Brandenberg Amethyst, Dumortierite, Gabbro, Kakortokite, Leopardskin Jasper, Pyrophyllite, Red Amethyst, Wind Fossil Agate

   dark night of: Golden Danburite, Khutnohorite, Stone of Sanctuary

   encrustations: Ethiopian Opal

   evolution: Hilulite, Paraiba Tourmaline, Shift Crystal

   growth: Agrellite, Beryllonite, Epidote

   healing: Amphibole, Black Kyanite, Blue Aragonite, Brandenberg Amethyst, Cassiterite, Ethiopian Opal,

Fiskenaesset Ruby, Khutnohorite, Marble, Nuummite, Pink Lazurine, Porphyrite (Chinese Letter Stone), Preseli Bluestone, Ruby Lavender Quartz, Trigonic Quartz

incarnate fully: Bushman Red Cascade Quartz, Celestial Quartz, Snakeskin Agate

imperatives: Nirvana Quartz, Porphyrite (Chinese Letter Stone), Tantalite

memory: Amphibole, Cacoxenite, Datolite, Trigonic Quartz

overcome fear in: Amphibole, Khutnohorite, Stone of Sanctuary, Revelation Stone, Tangerose

overlay: Scheelite

path/plan: Amblygonite, Anthrophyllite, Astrophyllite, Black Kyanite, Blue Aragonite, Brazilianite, Candle Quartz, Cathedral Quartz, Crystalline Kyanite, Datolite, Golden Danburite, Icicle Calcite, Indicolite Quartz, Khutnohorite, Lemurian Jade, Leopardskin Serpentine, Lepidocrosite, Merkabite Calcite, Paraiba Tourmaline, Rainbow Mayanite, Rainbow Moonstone, Stellar Beam Calcite

rescue: Tangerose

retrieval: Faden Quartz, Fulgarite, Epidote, Gaspeite, Khutnohorite, Mount Shasta Opal, Nuummite, Preseli Bluestone, Rainbow Mayanite, Snakeskin Agate, Tangerose. *Chakra:* higher heart, third eye

Soul Star chakra: see Chakras page 76

Unless otherwise directed, apply crystal over organ or site of symptom, place on appropriate chakra, wear as jewellery, bathe with or take as a crystal essence.

Sound healing, support: Libethenite, Smoky Amethyst

Spasms: Blue Aragonite, Diopside, Chrome Diopside, Malacholla, Pyrite in Magnesite

Speak out: Honey Opal, Titanite (Sphene), Xenotine. *Chakra:* throat

Speaking unthinkingly: Ethiopian Opal, Nzuri Moyo, Phosphosiderite. *Chakra:* base, throat

Speech impediments: Blue Crackle Quartz, Blue Euclase, Spider Web Obsidian. *Chakra:* third eye, throat

Spells, protection against: Larvikite, Master Shamanite, Owyhee Blue Opal, Nunderite, Nuummite, Purpurite, Tantalite. *Chakra:* throat, higher heart

Spinal:

  alignment: Blue Moonstone, Graphic Smoky Quartz (Zebra Stone), Huebnerite, Phantom Selenite, Scolecite, Shell Jasper, Stichtite, Tinguaite

  column: Calcite Fairy Stone, Huebnerite, Scolecite, Tinguaite

  inflexible: Blue Moonstone, Phantom Selenite, Scolecite, Tinguaite

  energy, blocked: Flame Aura Quartz, Garnet in Quartz, Strawberry Lemurian, Sedona Stone

  injuries: Cathedral Quartz

  out of alignment: Blue Moonstone, Graphic Smoky Quartz (Zebra Stone), Rainbow Moonstone, Scolecite, Vivianite, Tinguaite

  strengthen: Erythrite

Unless otherwise directed, apply crystal over organ or site of symptom, place on appropriate chakra, wear as jewellery, bathe with or take as a crystal essence.

Spiritual:

> **development:** Agnitite, Ajo Quartz, Anandalite, Andara Glass, Andescine Labradorite, Angels Wing Calcite, Auralite 23, Azeztulites of all types, Carolite, Celestobarite, Dianite, Eclipse Stone, Epiphany Quartz, Fire and Ice, Fire Obsidian, Firework Obsidian, Galaxyite, Glaucophane, Glendonite, Golden Coracalcite, Golden Healer, Green Ridge Quartz, Kambaba Jasper, Larvikite, Lodolite, Petrified Wood, Phlogopite, Prehnite with Epidote, Que Sera, Rainbow Mayanite, Ruby Lavender Quartz, Sedona Stone, Shell Jasper, Tantalite, Terraluminite, Titanite (Sphene), Violane
>
> > **blocked:** Auralite 23, Andara Glass, Bumble Bee Jasper, Celestobarite, Master Shamanite, Realgar, Rutilated Kunzite, Sedona Stone, Terraluminite, Titanite, Victorite
> >
> > **interference:** Mohawkite, Polychrome Jasper, Nunderite, Rainbow Mayanite, Tantalite. *Chakra:* crown (wear constantly)

Spirit release: Nirvana Quartz and see Entity release page 106

Spleen: Aegirine, Apple Aura Quartz, Black Moonstone, Blue Quartz, Brochantite, Bustamite, Cinnabar in Jasper, Guinea Fowl Jasper, Marcasite, Nunderite, Orange River Quartz. *Chakra:* spleen

> **blood flow:** Mookaite Jasper

Unless otherwise directed, apply crystal over organ or site of symptom, place on appropriate chakra, wear as jewellery, bathe with or take as a crystal essence.

deterioration: Mookaite Jasper, Prasiolite

detoxifying: Amechlorite, Banded Agate, Eye of the Storm, Jamesonite, Larvikite, Pyrite in Magnesite, Rainbow Covellite, Richterite, Smoky Quartz with Aegerine, Shungite

protection: Nunderite, Tugtupite

Spleen chakra: see Chakras pages 76–82

Sports injuries: Aegirine, Blue Moonstone, Dream Quartz and see also Muscles page 150

Sprains: Dalmatian Stone, Dream Quartz, Epidote, Gabbro

Stability: Celestobarite, Eye of the Storm, Smoky Elestial Quartz. *Chakra:* base, dantien

Stage fright: Dumortierite

Stagnant energy: Chrome Diopside, Eye of the Storm, Garnet in Quartz, Poppy Jasper, Ruby Lavender Quartz, Sedona Stone, Shaman Quartz, Tantalite and see Negative energy page 152. *Chakra:* base, dantien

Stamina: Anthrophyllite, Epidote, Purpurite. *Chakra:* base, dantien

Stammering: Greenlandite. *Chakra:* throat, third eye

Star children: Fairy Quartz, Calcite Fairy Stone, Empowerite, Glaucophane, Star Hollandite, Starseed Quartz. *Chakra:* higher crown

Star being, contact: Aswan Granite, Glaucophane, Lemurian Seed, Scolecite, Star Hollandite, Mount Shasta Opal, Scolecite, Starseed Quartz, Sugar Blade Quartz

Unless otherwise directed, apply crystal over organ or site of symptom, place on appropriate chakra, wear as jewellery, bathe with or take as a crystal essence.

Stellar Gateway chakra: see Chakras page 76

Steroids, boosting natural: Poppy Jasper. *Chakra:* higher heart, dantien

Stiff neck: Alexandrite. *Chakra:* throat

Stitches: Stichtite

Stomach: Amblygonite, Black Moonstone, Bytownite, Bismuth, Cryolite, Mookaite Jasper, Paraiba Tourmaline, Prasiolite, Serpentine in Obsidian, Snakeskin Agate, Stibnite, Turritella Agate, Tugtupite. *Chakra:* solar plexus

    acidity: Barite, Bismuth, Kimberlite, Snakeskin Agate

    cramps: Bastnasite, Cat's Eye Quartz, Orange Moss Agate, Serpentine in Obsidian, Zircon

    problems as a result of stress: Amechlorite, Barite, Bird's Eye Jasper, Eisenkiesel, Eye of the Storm, Marble, Riebekite with Sugilite and Bustamite, Shungite

    swollen: Barite

    ulcer: Blue Siberian Quartz, Hemimorphite

Strained muscles: Aegirine, Blue Moonstone, Diopside (and see Muscles page 150)

Streptococcal infections: Malacholla, Shungite (wear over throat and take crystal essence frequently)

Stress: Andean Blue Opal, Atlantasite, Basalt, Bird's Eye Jasper, Bronzite, Dumortierite, Cacoxenite, Eisenkiesel, Eye of the Storm, Gabbro, Green Diopside, Hematoid Calcite, Marble, Mariposite, Mount Shasta Opal, Nuummite, Ocean Jasper, Paraiba Tourmaline, Pyrite in

Magnesite, Red Amethyst, Richterite, Riebekite with Sugilite and Bustamite, Shungite

> **related illness:** Ajoite with Shattuckite, Amechlorite, Blue Aragonite, Blue Siberian Quartz, Bustamite, Candle Quartz, Epidote, Fiskenaesset Ruby, Morion, Mount Shasta Opal, Quantum Quattro, Riebekite with Sugilite and Bustamite. *Chakra:* third eye, heart, solar plexus

Stretch marks: Stichtite

Stroke damage: Black Moonstone, Clevelandite

Subconscious blocks: Lepidocrosite, Molybdenite in Quartz, Smoky Elestial Quartz, Smoky Spirit Quartz. *Chakra:* dantien

Subtle bodies: see Aura page 58 and Lightbody page 137

Suicidal tendencies: Brandenberg Amethyst, Pink Petalite (wear constantly)

Sun sensitivity: Lazulite

Sunburn: Blue Siberian Quartz, Dumortierite, Lazulite

Supra-adrenals: Axinite, Cacoxenite, Epidote, Eye of the Storm, Gaspeite, Nunderite, Picrolite, Richterite. *Chakra:* dantien (or tape over kidneys)

Superiority: Heulandite. *Chakra:* dantien

Suppurating wounds: Diaspore (Zultanite), Klinoptilolith, Schalenblende, Shungite

Surgery, recovery: Brookite, Eisenkiesel, Empowerite, Enstatite and Diopside, Eye of the Storm, Fire Obsidian, Green Diopside, Stromatolite

---

Unless otherwise directed, apply crystal over organ or site of symptom, place on appropriate chakra, wear as jewellery, bathe with or take as a crystal essence.

Survival instincts: Ammolite, Kimberlite, Thunder Egg.
Chakra: base

Sweats: Indicolite Quartz, Menalite

Swelling: Agrellite, Anandalite™, Andean Blue Opal, Blue Euclase, Bornite, Chinese Red Quartz, Crystal Cap Amethyst, Smoky Amethyst

Swollen:

    feet: Andean Blue Opal

    glands and lymphatics: Agrellite, Smoky Amethyst, Shungite and see lymphatics page 141

    joints: Bastnasite, Andean Blue Opal, Smoky Amethyst and see joints page 131

Unless otherwise directed, apply crystal over organ or site of symptom, place on appropriate chakra, wear as jewellery, bathe with or take as a crystal essence.

- T -

Tachycardia: Ammolite, Purpurite. *Chakra:* dantien, heart

Taking on other people's feelings or conditions: Brochantite, Healer's Gold, Iridescent Pyrite, Lemurian Jade, Mohawkite. *Chakra:* solar plexus, spleen

Tantric practices: Anandalite™, Eudialyte, Kundalini Quartz, Serpentine in Obsidian, Tiffany Stone, Victorite

Taste, loss of: Mystic Topaz

T-cells: Diaspore (Zultanite), Klinoptilolith, Quantum Quattro, Que Sera, Richterite, Rosophia, Tangerine Sun Aura Quartz, Tangerose. *Chakra:* higher heart

Teeth: Brookite, Cavansite, Fluorapatite, Glendonite, Molybdenite, Paraiba Tourmaline, Phlogopite, Poldervaarite, Pyrite in Magnesite, Shell Jasper, Stichtite, Stromatolite, Strontianite, Titanite (Sphene), Winchite, Wind Fossil Agate

    enamel: Phlogopite, Strontianite

    mercury amalgam, antidote: Brazilianite, Chinese Chromium Quartz, Que Sera

Teething pain: Blue Euclase, Cathedral Quartz, Quantum Quattro, Rhodozite

Telepathy: Afghanite, Arsenopyrite, Auralite 23, Avalonite, Blue Selenite, Blue Siberian Quartz, Eilat Stone, Limonite, Red Amethyst, Sichuan Quartz, Tanzanite

Unless otherwise directed, apply crystal over organ or site of symptom, place on appropriate chakra, wear as jewellery, bathe with or take as a crystal essence.

Temperature, regulate: Crackled Fire Agate, Dinosaur Bone, Nuummite, Pyrite in Magnesite (place beside left ear)

Temper tantrums: Neptunite, Pearl Spa Dolomite. *Chakra:* base, dantien

Tendonitis: Rosophia, Steatite, Strontianite, Tiffany Stone

Tension, release: Green Ridge Quartz, Mystic Topaz, Star Hollandite, Strawberry Quartz. *Chakra:* base, heart, solar plexus

Terminal illness, support during: Diopside, Eye of the Storm, Sonora Sunrise, Tangerose, Tremolite, Winchite

Testicles: see Reproductive system page 177

Theta brainwaves: see Brain page 69

Thought form, disperse: Aegerine, Firework Obsidian, Nuummite, Rainbow Mayanite, Scolecite, Smoky Amethyst, Smoky Citrine, Spectrolite, Stibnite

Thoughts racing: Auralite 23, Blue Selenite, Pearl Spa Dolomite, Rhomboid Calcite, Scolecite

Third eye (brow chakra): see Chakras pages 76 and 82

Throat: Blue Quartz, Blue Siberian Quartz, Chrysotile, Chrysotile in Serpentine, Eclipse Stone, Glaucophane, Indicolite Quartz, Owyhee Blue Opal, Paraiba Tourmaline, Stromatolite. *Chakra:* third eye

   chakra: see pages 76 and 82

   infected: Owyhee Blue Opal, Shungite (gargle)

   inflamed: Alexandrite, Blue Euclase, Blue Siberian

Unless otherwise directed, apply crystal over organ or site of symptom, place on appropriate chakra, wear as jewellery, bathe with or take as a crystal essence.

Quartz, Hanksite, Indicolite Quartz, Owyhee Blue Opal, Shungite

sore: Indicolite Quartz, Paraiba Tourmaline

ulcerated: Hemimorphite, Owyhee Blue Opal

Thrombosis: see Blood clots page 65

Thrush: Dendritic Chalcedony, Shungite

Thymus: Andean Opal, Chrysotile, Eilat Stone, Blue Halite, Indicolite Quartz, Prehnite with Epidote, Quantum Quattro, Que Sera, Richterite, Shaman Quartz, Stromatolite, Thompsonite, Tremolite. *Chakra:* higher heart

underactive: Eilat Stone

Thyroid: Blue Halite, Champagne Aura Quartz, Cryolite, Cumberlandite, Eilat Stone, Indicolite Quartz, Lazulite, Leopardskin Serpentine, Paraiba Tourmaline, Prehnite with Epidote, Quantum Quattro, Richterite, Tanzine Aura Quartz. *Chakra:* throat

deficiencies: Tanzine Aura Quartz

balance: Cacoxenite, Richterite

regulate: Tanzine Aura Quartz, Richterite

stimulate: Tanzine Aura Quartz

Tics: Fenster Quartz and see Twitches page 130

Tie cutting: Flint, Leopardskin Jasper, Novaculite, Rainbow Mayanite, Stibnite

Tinnitus: Ammolite, Dogtooth Calcite, Ocean Jasper, Peanut Wood, Serpentine, Xenotine

Tiredness: Poppy Jasper, Purpurite and see Fatigue page

110. *Chakra:* base, dantien

Tissue:

    connective: Greenlandite, Desert Rose, Piemontite, Prehnite with Epidote

    degeneration: Alexandrite, Eilat Stone, Tantalite

    detoxify: Amechlorite, Eye of the Storm, Fairy Quartz, Jamesonite, Larvikite, Phlogopite, Pyrite in Magnesite, Rainbow Covellite, Richterite, Shungite, Smoky Amethyst, Smoky Quartz with Aegerine, Tantalite

    hardened: Prehnite with Epidote, Pumice

    repair: Alexandrite, Diaspore (Zultanite), Eilat Stone, Eisenkiesel, Greenlandite, Flint, Khutnohorite, Piemontite, Tantalite

    regeneration: Alexandrite, Eilat Stone, Flint, Leopardskin Jasper, Nuummite, Tantalite

    torn: Creedite, Eisenkiesel, Khutnohorite, Phlogopite, Piemontite, Tantalite

Toenails, fungal infections: Covellite, Klinoptilolith, Rainbow Covellite, Shungite

Tonic: Quantum Quattro, Que Sera, Poppy Jasper

Tonsillitis: Indicolite Quartz, Quantum Quattro, Shungite. *Chakra:* base

Tonsils, inflamed: Indicolite Quartz, Shungite. *Chakra:* base

Toxic earth meridians: Granite, Kambaba Jasper, Mohawkite, Smoky Elestial Quartz, Snakeskin Pyrite,

Valentinite and Stibnite

Toxicity: Arsenopyrite, Champagne Aura Quartz, Klinoptilolith, Morion Quartz, Smoky Quartz Elestial, Snakeskin Pyrite, Valentinite and Stibnite. *Chakra:* dantien

Toothache: Cathedral Quartz, Quantum Quattro, Shungite

Tourette's syndrome: Fenster Quartz

Toxins: see Detoxification page 95. *Chakra:* earth star, spleen

> **disperse:** Actinolite, Aegerine, Banded Agate, Barite, Blue Quartz, Celestobarite, Champagne Aura Quartz, Chinese Chromium Quartz, Conichalcite, Covellite, Golden Danburite, Danburite with Chlorite, Eilat Stone, Epidote, Eye of the Storm, Fairy Quartz, Fiskenaesset Ruby, Halite, Hanksite, Huebnerite, Leopardskin Serpentine, Morion, Ocean Jasper, Pearl Spa Dolomite, Poppy Jasper, Pumice, Pyrite in Quartz, Quantum Quattro, Smoky Elestial Quartz, Smoky Herkimer, Snakeskin Pyrite, Spirit Quartz. *Chakra:* base, earth star, dantien, spleen, solar plexus
>
> **strengthen resistance to:** Eye of the Storm, Klinoptilolith, Ocean Jasper, Pyrite in Quartz, Shungite. *Chakra:* base, earth star, dantien, spleen, solar plexus

Tranquillizer: Amblygonite, Blue Quartz, Candle Quartz, Leopardskin Jasper, Poppy Jasper, Pounamou

---

Unless otherwise directed, apply crystal over organ or site of symptom, place on appropriate chakra, wear as jewellery, bathe with or take as a crystal essence.

Jade, Quantum Quattro, Strawberry Quartz, Vera Cruz Amethyst. *Chakra:* higher heart

Transition: Arfvedsonite, Crocoite, Lemurian Jade, Peach Selenite, Rhodozite, Smoky Lemurian, Smoky Spirit Quartz

Trauma: Ammolite, Blue Euclase, Bornite, Brandenberg Amethyst, Cathedral Quartz, Cavansite, Empowerite, Garnet in Quartz, Green Diopside, Dumortierite, Epidote, Faden Quartz, Fulgarite, Gaia Stone, Goethite, Green Ridge Quartz, Guardian Stone, Kimberlite, Mangano Vesuvianite, Novaculite with Nuummite, Ocean Blue Jasper, Oregon Opal, Peach Selenite, Peanut Wood, Prasiolite, Richterite, Ruby Lavender Quartz, Scapolite, Sea Sediment Jasper, Smoky Elestial, Spirit Quartz, Tantalite, Victorite, Wavellite, Youngite. *Chakra:* solar plexus (or wear constantly)

Travel sickness: Aztee, Gaspeite

Traveller's diarrhoea: Libyan Gold Tektite. *Chakra:* dantien

Triple burner meridian, rebalance: Crackled Fire Agate, Nuummite (place beside left ear)

Truth, speak: Astraline. *Chakra:* throat

Tuberculosis: Graphic Smoky Quartz (Zebra Stone)

Tumours: Annabergite, Champagne Aura Quartz, Covellite, Eilat Stone, Fluorapatite, Gabbro, Klinoptilolith, Lepidocrosite, Ocean Jasper, Ouro Verde, Prasiolite, Uranophane (under supervision)

Unless otherwise directed, apply crystal over organ or site of symptom, place on appropriate chakra, wear as jewellery, bathe with or take as a crystal essence.

asbestos related: Actinolite
Typhoid fever: Holly Agate. *Chakra:* dantien

- U -

Ulcers: Blue Siberian Quartz, Cryolite, Hemimorphite, Montebrasite, Quantum Quattro

    eyes: Vivianite

    intestinal: Bismuth, Gaspeite, Honey Calcite

    stomach: Blue Siberian Quartz

    varicose: Bastnasite, Marialite, Prophecy Stone, Scapolite

Unacceptable thoughts and feelings: Scolecite, Vivianite. *Chakra:* solar plexus, third eye

Unconditional love: Astraline, Cobalto Calcite, Tangerose, Tugtupite. *Chakra:* higher heart (wear continuously or place over higher heart)

Ungroundedness: Aztee, Basalt, Celestobarite, Dragon Stone, Empowerite, Granite, Graphic Smoky Quartz (Zebra Stone), Kambaba Jasper, Mohawkite, Peanut Wood, Polychrome Jasper, Proustite, Serpentine in Obsidian, Shell Jasper, Smoky Elestial Quartz, Steatite, Stromatolite. *Chakra:* earth star, base, dantien (or place behind knees)

Upset stomach with headache: Dumortierite, Rhodozite

Urethra: Scheelite

Urogenital tract: Black Kyanite, Scheelite, Violane. *Chakra:* sacral, dantien

Urinary tract infections: Bastnasite, Fire and Ice Quartz, Richterite

---

Unless otherwise directed, apply crystal over organ or site of symptom, place on appropriate chakra, wear as jewellery, bathe with or take as a crystal essence.

Uterus: Menalite, Shiva Lingam. *Chakra:* sacral
Uterine bleeding: Flint, Menalite. *Chakra:* sacral

Unless otherwise directed, apply crystal over organ or site of symptom, place on appropriate chakra, wear as jewellery, bathe with or take as a crystal essence.

- V -

Vacillation: Brucite. *Chakra:* dantien

Vagina: Shiva Lingam. *Chakra:* sacral

Vampirism of heart energy: Gaspeite, Greenlandite, Iridescent Pyrite, Lemurian Aquitane Calcite, Nunderite, Tantalite, Xenotine. *Chakra:* solar plexus, heart, higher heart

Vampirism of spleen energy: Gaspeite, Iridescent Pyrite, Nunderite, Tantalite, Xenotine. *Chakra:* spleen

Vascular cramps: Bastnasite, Cat's Eye Quartz, Orange Moss Agate, Pyrite in Magnesite, Serpentine in Obsidian

Veins: Benitoite, Chohua Jasper, Chrysotile, Goethite, Graphic Smoky Quartz (Zebra Stone), Mangano Vesuvianite, Rainbow Moonstone

> **thread:** Chalcopyrite
>
> **varicose:** Scapolite

Venomous bites: Shungite

Vertebrae: see Spinal page 187

Vertigo: Celestobarite, Dogtooth Calcite, Fairy Quartz, Zircon (place on back of neck)

Vibrational change, facilitate: Anandalite, Bismuth, Gabbro, Huebnerite, Lemurian Gold Opal, Lemurian Jade, Luxullianite, Montebrasite, Mtrolite, Nunderite, Rainbow Mayanite, Rosophia, Sanda Rosa Azeztulite, Snakeskin Pyrite, Sonora Sunrise, Trigonic Quartz. *Chakra:* higher heart, higher crown (wear stones

---

Unless otherwise directed, apply crystal over organ or site of symptom, place on appropriate chakra, wear as jewellery, bathe with or take as a crystal essence.

frequently or keep within reach and hold frequently)

Victim mentality: Amblygonite, Brazilianite, Epidote, Green Ridge Quartz, Hematoid Calcite, Ice Quartz, Marcasite, Orange River Quartz, Smoky Lemurian Seed, Tugtupite with Nuummite, Zircon. *Chakra:* dantien

Violence, negate: Eye of the Storm (Judy's Jasper). *Chakra:* base (keep in environment)

Viral infections: Cathedral Quartz, Himalayan Red Azeztulite, Proustite, Rainforest Jasper, Shaman Quartz, Shungite. *Chakra:* higher heart

Virility, increase: Poppy Jasper. *Chakra:* base, sacral, dantien

Vision: Holey Stone, Mystic Topaz and see Eyes page 108

Vitality, increase: Crackled Fire Agate, Eye of the Storm, Larvikite, Quantum Quattro, Que Sera, Poppy Jasper, Pyrite in Quartz, Red Chohua Jasper, Rhodozite, Ruby in Granite, Sedona Stone, Sonora Sunrise, Strontianite. *Chakra:* base

Vitamin, non-absorption: Orchid Calcite, and see Assimilation page 56. *Chakra:* solar plexus

Vocal cords: Blue Aragonite, Hackmanite, Indicolite Quartz, Lemurian Aquitane Calcite, Owyhee Blue Opal. *Chakra:* throat (wear or take crystal essence)

Voice work: Blue Aragonite

Vomiting: Dumortierite, Gaspeite, Green Calcite. *Chakra:* solar plexus

Vulnerability: Tangerose

Unless otherwise directed, apply crystal over organ or site of symptom, place on appropriate chakra, wear as jewellery, bathe with or take as a crystal essence.

- W -

Warts: Flint, Hemimorphite, Snakeskin Agate

Walking difficulties: Peanut Wood

War zones: Afghanite, Eye of the Storm (Judy's Jasper), Tanzanite

Wasting disorders: Dumortierite

Water purifier: Shungite (leave in water for 24–48 hours)

Water retention: Andean Blue Opal, Bustamite, Halite, Hanksite. *Chakra:* dantien

Weak:

> **energy field:** Chrome Diopside, Quantum Quattro, Que Sera, Poppy Jasper, Sedona Stone (hold between sacral and solar plexus)
>
> **muscles:** Blue Moonstone and see Muscles page 150

Weather sensitivity: Avalonite, Golden Pietersite. *Chakra:* third eye

Well-being, promote: Beryllonite, Fiskenaesset Ruby, Fulgarite, Ice Quartz, Keyiapo, Shift Crystal, Strawberry Quartz, Tugtupite, Ussingite. *Chakra:* higher heart

Weight:

> **causes behind:** Epidote, Ethiopian Opal, Heulandite
>
> **control:** Chinese Chromium Quartz, Drusy Golden Healer, Diaspore (Zultanite)
>
> **loss:** Diaspore (Zultanite), Hemimorphite, Heulandite, Pearl Spa Dolomite, Picasso Jasper, Peanut Wood

---

Unless otherwise directed, apply crystal over organ or site of symptom, place on appropriate chakra, wear as jewellery, bathe with or take as a crystal essence.

over: Chinese Chromium Quartz, Ethiopian Opal, Hemimorphite

under: see Anorexia page 55

White cell count: Wavellite

Willpower: Cat's Eye Quartz, Gold Siberian Quartz, Marcasite, Montebrasite, Preseli Bluestone, Silver Leaf Jasper. *Chakra:* base, dantien

Will to be cured: Golden Healer Quartz. *Chakra:* dantien

Wisdom: Amphibole Quartz, Atlantasite, Avalonite, Bytownite, Calligraphy Stone, Cathedral Quartz, Chrysotile, Covellite, Creedite, Dumortierite, Golden Danburite, Golden Herkimer, Eilat Stone, Greenlandite, Hanksite, Lemurian Seed, Leopardskin Jasper, Libyan Gold Tektite, Merlinite, Nirvana Quartz, Ouro Verde, Paraiba Tourmaline, Peach Selenite, Ocean Jasper, Sichuan Quartz, Spectrolite, Star Hollandite, Starseed Quartz, Stellar Beam Calcite, Tibetan Black Spot Quartz, Trigonic Quartz, Ussingite. *Chakra:* crown

Worry, excessive: Pink Crackle Quartz, Revelation Stone, Snakeskin Agate, Sonora Sunrise

Workplace: Amphibole, Candle Quartz, Hematoid Calcite, Spirit Quartz

Wounds: Ajoite, Andean Blue Opal, Atlantasite, Bixbite, Diaspore (Zultanite), Flint, Gaia Stone, Klinoptilolith, Mookaite Jasper, Pumice, Quantum Quattro, Schalenblende, Seriphos Quartz, Shungite, Youngite

Wrinkles, remove: Flint, Riebekite with Sugilite and

Bustamite, Snakeskin Agate (bathe skin in crystal essence)

Writer's block: Agrellite, Calligraphy Stone, Chinese Writing Stone, Crackled Fire Agate, Valentinite and Stibnite. *Chakra:* dantien

Unless otherwise directed, apply crystal over organ or site of symptom, place on appropriate chakra, wear as jewellery, bathe with or take as a crystal essence.

- X -

X-rays, prevent damage from: Black Moonstone, Smoky Elestial Quartz, Smoky Herkimer, Shungite (wear constantly, rub crystal essence over site, take crystal essence frequently), Torbernite (use under supervision)

- Y -

Yin-yang imbalances: Alunite, Dalmatian Stone, Day and Night Quartz, Eilat Stone, Poppy Jasper, Morion, Scheelite, Shiva Lingam. *Chakra:* base, dantien

- Z -

Zest for life: Bushman Red Cascade, Orange River Quartz, Poppy Jasper, Zebra Stone. *Chakra:* dantien
Zinc absorption: Pyrite in Sphalerite. *Chakra:* solar plexus

---

Unless otherwise directed, apply crystal over organ or site of symptom, place on appropriate chakra, wear as jewellery, bathe with or take as a crystal essence.

Resources

Crystal suppliers

Crystals specially charged for you by Judy Hall are available at www.angeladditions.co.uk

High vibration crystals in the UK are available from www.hehishelo.co.uk and www.ksccrystals.com

Excellent high vibration crystals in the States are available from www.exquisitecrystals.com and www.neatstuff.net/avalon

Crystal cleansers

Clear 2 Light from www.petaltone.co.uk is an excellent crystal cleanser and is available worldwide. Crystal Charge is also available from Petaltone.

Crystal Cleanser spray from the Crystal Balance Company and Crystal Recharge along with transmuting Violet Flame work wonders (www.crystalbalance.net).

Further reading by Judy Hall

Hall, Judy, *Crystal Prescriptions 1* (O-Books, Alresford, 2005)

Hall, Judy, *Crystal Bibles, vols 1–3* (Godsfield Press, London, UK; Walking Stick Press, USA)

Hall, Judy, *Earth Blessings: Using Crystals for Personal Energy Clearing, Earth Healing and Environmental Enhancement* (Watkins Books, London, 2014)

Hall, Judy *101 Power Crystals: The Ultimate Guide to Magical Crystals, Gems, and Stones for Healing and Transformation* (Fair Winds, USA; Quarto, London)

Hall, Judy *The Crystal Healing Pack* (Godsfield, London)

Hall, Judy *Crystals and Sacred Sites: Use Crystals to Access the Power of Sacred Landscapes for Personal and Planetary Transformation* (Fair Winds, USA, 2012)

Hall, Judy *The Crystal Experience: Your Complete Crystal Workshop in a Book* (Godsfield, London, 2012)

Hall, Judy *The Encyclopedia of Crystals* (Godsfield Press, Fair Winds, USA, revised edition 2013)

Hall, Judy, *Psychic Self-Protection: Using Crystals to Change Your Life* (Hay House)

Hall, Judy, *Good Vibrations: Psychic Protection, Energy Enhancement, Space Clearing* (Flying Horse Publications, Bournemouth)

Hall, Judy, *Life Changing Crystals: Using crystals to manifest abundance, wellbeing and happiness* (Godsfield Press, UK, 2013); *Crystals to Empower You* (F&W, USA, 2013)

Hall, Judy, *The Crystal Wisdom Oracle* (Watkins Books, London, 2013)

Volumes in this series:

Crystal Prescriptions

The A–Z guide to over 1,200 symptoms and their healing
crystals
ISBN: 978-1-90504-740-6 (Paperback) £7.99 $15.95

Crystal Prescriptions volume 3

Crystal solutions to electromagnetic pollution and geopathic
stress. An A–Z guide.
ISBN: 978-1-78279-791-3 (Paperback) £8.99 $14.95

Crystal Prescriptions volume 4

The A–Z guide to the chakra balancing crystals and kundalini
activation stones
ISBN: 978-1-78535-053-5 (Paperback) £10.99 $17.95

Crystal Prescriptions volume 5

Space clearing, Feng Shui and Psychic Protection.
An A-Z guide.
ISBN: 978-1-78535-457-1 (Paperback) £12.99 $19.95

Crystal Prescriptions volume 6

Crystals for ancestral clearing, soul retrieval, spirit release and
karmic healing. An A-Z guide.
ISBN: 978-1-78535-455-7 (Paperback) £13.99 $19.95

Crystal Prescriptions volume 7

The A–Z guide to creating crystal essences for abundant
well-being, environmental healing and astral-magic
ISBN: 978-1-78904-052-4 (Paperback) £14.99 $23.95

BOOKS

O-BOOKS

SPIRITUALITY

O is a symbol of the world, of oneness and unity; this eye represents knowledge and insight. We publish titles on general spirituality and living a spiritual life. We aim to inform and help you on your own journey in this life. If you have enjoyed this book, why not tell other readers by posting a review on your preferred book site?

Recent bestsellers from O-Books are:

Heart of Tantric Sex

Diana Richardson

Revealing Eastern secrets of deep love and intimacy to
Western couples.

Paperback: 978-1-90381-637-0 ebook: 978-1-84694-637-0

Crystal Prescriptions

The A-Z guide to over 1,200 symptoms and their healing
crystals

Judy Hall

The first in the popular series of eight books, this handy
little guide is packed as tight as a pill-bottle with crystal
remedies for ailments.

Paperback: 978-1-90504-740-6 ebook: 978-1-84694-629-5

Take Me To Truth

Undoing the Ego

Nouk Sanchez, Tomas Vieira

The best-selling step-by-step book on shedding the Ego,
using the teachings of *A Course In Miracles*.

Paperback: 978-1-84694-050-7 ebook: 978-1-84694-654-7

The 7 Myths about Love...Actually!

The journey from your HEAD to the HEART of your SOUL

Mike George

Smashes all the myths about LOVE.

Paperback: 978-1-84694-288-4 ebook: 978-1-84694-682-0

The Holy Spirit's Interpretation of the New Testament
A Course in Understanding and Acceptance
Regina Dawn Akers
Following on from the strength of *A Course In Miracles*,
NTI teaches us how to experience the love and oneness
of God.
Paperback: 978-1-84694-085-9 ebook: 978-1-78099-083-5

The Message of A Course In Miracles
A translation of the text in plain language
Elizabeth A. Cronkhite
A translation of *A Course in Miracles* into plain, everyday
language for anyone seeking inner peace. The
companion volume, *Practicing A Course In Miracles*,
offers practical lessons and mentoring.
Paperback: 978-1-84694-319-5 ebook: 978-1-84694-642-4

Thinker's Guide to God
Peter Vardy
An introduction to key issues in the philosophy of
religion.
Paperback: 978-1-90381-622-6

Your Simple Path
Find happiness in every step
Ian Tucker
A guide to helping us reconnect with what is really
important in our lives.
Paperback: 978-1-78279-349-6 ebook: 978-1-78279-348-9

365 Days of Wisdom
Daily Messages To Inspire You Through The Year
Dadi Janki
Daily messages which cool the mind, warm the heart
and guide you along your journey.
Paperback: 978-1-84694-863-3 ebook: 978-1-84694-864-0

Body of Wisdom
Women's Spiritual Power and How it Serves
Hilary Hart
Bringing together the dreams and experiences of women
across the world with today's most visionary spiritual
teachers.
Paperback: 978-1-78099-696-7 ebook: 978-1-78099-695-0

Dying to Be Free
From Enforced Secrecy to Near Death to True
Transformation
Hannah Robinson
After an unexpected accident and near-death
experience, Hannah Robinson found herself radically
transforming her life, while a remarkable new insight
altered her relationship with her father a practising
Catholic priest.
Paperback: 978-1-78535-254-6 ebook: 978-1-78535-255-3

The Ecology of the Soul
A Manual of Peace, Power and Personal Growth for Real
People in the Real World
Aidan Walker
Balance your own inner Ecology of the Soul to regain
your natural state of peace, power and wellbeing.
Paperback: 978-1-78279-850-7 ebook: 978-1-78279-849-1

Not I, Not other than I
The Life and Teachings of Russel Williams
Steve Taylor, Russel Williams
The miraculous life and inspiring teachings of one of the
World's greatest living Sages.
Paperback: 978-1-78279-729-6 ebook: 978-1-78279-728-9

On the Other Side of Love
A Woman's Unconventional Journey Towards Wisdom
Muriel Maufroy
When life has lost all meaning, what do you do?
Paperback: 978-1-78535-281-2 ebook: 978-1-78535-282-9

Practicing A Course In Miracles
A Translation of the Workbook in Plain Language and
With Mentoring Notes
Elizabeth A. Cronkhite
The practical second and third volumes of The Plain-
Language *A Course In Miracles*.
Paperback: 978-1-84694-403-1 ebook: 978-1-78099-072-9

Quantum Bliss
The Quantum Mechanics of Happiness, Abundance, and
Health
George S. Mentz
Quantum Bliss is the breakthrough summary of success
and spirituality secrets that customers have been
waiting for.
Paperback: 978-1-78535-203-4 ebook: 978-1-78535-204-1

The Upside Down Mountain
Mags MacKean
A must-read for anyone weary of chasing success and
happiness – one woman's inspirational journey
swapping the uphill slog for the downhill slope.
Paperback: 978-1-78535-171-6 ebook: 978-1-78535-172-3

Your Personal Tuning Fork
The Endocrine System
Deborah Bates
Discover your body's health secret, the endocrine
system, and 'twang' your way to sustainable health!
Paperback: 978-1-84694-503-8 ebook: 978-1-78099-697-4